COME HOME ALIVE

THE POWER OF KNOWING HOW TO WORK TOGETHER TO MAKE IT THROUGH THE CRISIS OF CANCER

MARI D. MARTIN

WESTBOW
P R E S S®
A DIVISION OF THOMAS NELSON
& ZONDERVAN

WestBow Press books may be ordered through booksellers or by contacting:

WestBow Press
A Division of Thomas Nelson & Zondervan
1663 Liberty Drive
Bloomington, IN 47403
www.westbowpress.com
844-714-3454

Laura Veldhof Designs. LLC (Author Photo)
Rob Walcott Photography
© 2020 Kathy Kolbe and Kolbe Corp. All Rights Reserved 2020
Expect a Miracle Home (Lake Geneva) Website

ISBN: 978-1-6642-2299-1 (sc)
ISBN: 978-1-6642-2300-4 (hc)
ISBN: 978-1-6642-2298-4 (e)

Library of Congress Control Number: 2021902711

Print information available on the last page.

WestBow Press rev. date: 03/26/2021

This book is dedicated to my sister, Monica, who believed her sole purpose in life was to care for her husband, Dr. Edward Morris (1933–2017), when he could no longer care for himself.

CONTENTS

Foreword..ix

PART 1: INSPIRATION

Chapter 1   Inspiration 1
Chapter 2   Words Matter 4
Chapter 3   Running Renegade 7
Chapter 4   Diagnosis... 13
Chapter 5   Ticking Time Bomb... 17
Chapter 6   Light for the Way They Should Take...................... 20
Chapter 7   Do Not Be Afraid... 25
Chapter 8   Phone Home 27
Chapter 9   The Gift of Presence.. 29

PART 2: PRAYER

Chapter 10   Prayer 37
Chapter 11   My Prayer Focus... 43

PART 3: BELIEVE

Chapter 12   We Believe 51
Chapter 13   You Are Not a Doctor.. 59
Chapter 14   Hospital 63

PART 4: KNOW THE PATIENT

Chapter 15   Thriving to Heal 69
Chapter 16   Kolbe Is a Breakthrough 74
Chapter 17   Acting on What You Know.............................. 81
Chapter 18   Unknowns, Ambiguities, Complications 83
Chapter 19   The Lifeline of Humility 87

PART 5: KNOW THE CAREGIVER

Chapter 20   Know Your Modus Operandi (MO)............................ 95
Chapter 21   Who Is in Your Boat? 100
Chapter 22   In Relationship 104
Chapter 23   Do Not Die of Caregiving................................112
Chapter 24   Decision Fatigue 115
Chapter 25   This Could Go Either Way................................118
Chapter 26   Troubling Symptoms 120
Chapter 27   Words and Actions Really Matter............................ 122
Chapter 28   Words That Encourage 125
Chapter 29   Just Between You and Me............................... 126
Chapter 30   I Run to Hear.. 128
Chapter 31   What I Have Learned about Cancer 134

PART 6: BE GRATEFUL AND THANKFUL

Chapter 32   Be Grateful and Thankful................................141
Chapter 33   Presence in Action.................................... 146

PART 7: EXPECT A MIRACLE

Chapter 34   Do You Believe in Miracles?.............................151
Chapter 35   Time Line of a Miracle............................... 155
Chapter 36   The Miracle of New Life.............................. 164
Chapter 37   The Miracle of a Healing Practice 166
Chapter 38   The Miracle of Love...................................169

PART 8: WE WAIT

Chapter 39 Chicago Marathon 2017 175
Chapter 40 Pretty Well 184
Chapter 41 Faith through Affliction 187
Chapter 42 Come Home Alive 189

PART 9: CALL TO ACTION

Chapter 43 Call to Action... 195

Afterword 201
Disclaimer Page... 203
Acknowledgments.. 205
Notes 207
Recommended Reading 219
Training, Coaching, Consulting, and Speaking Services.............. 223

FOREWORD

For years, Mari Martin has shared her highly professional expertise for the sake of helping her clients grow in positive ways. Here, she has shared her highly personal journey for those who are evolving in more personal ways.

Readers may find themselves comparing parallel experiences from which she developed effective approaches for both acceptance and persistence. Mari gives us a practicum in taking on gut-wrenching problems by building a set of both reliable and relatable "tools." Then she shared how they've tied to the development of her beliefs.

Her journey, while personal, is meant to be universal. Her style is very accessible. Who among us dare review our own—let alone another's—emotion-driven decisions? She shows no need to second-guess herself; nor is the reader inclined to do so.

Perseverance in detailing her pain would be expected of this author. Being persuasive in describing the process as being inspiring takes it to another level.

Mari providing this book now is a blessing for many who will benefit from her sharing her fears, worries, and frustrations. She gives hope through descriptions of the paths she's found amiable, sensible, and inspiring. For many readers, this is exactly what's needed.

—Kathy Kolbe
Founder, Kolbe Corp.
Scottsdale, Arizona

Be on your guard;
stand firm in the faith;
be men of courage;
be strong.

1 Corinthians 16:13

PART 1

INSPIRATION

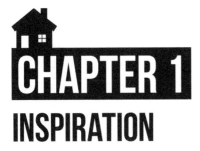

CHAPTER 1

INSPIRATION

*Indeed he was ill and almost died. But God had
mercy on him, and not on him only but also
on me, to spare me sorrow upon sorrow.*
—*Philippians 2:27*

*So Abraham called that place The Lord Will
Provide. And to this day it is said, "On the
mountain of the Lord it will be provided."*
—*Genesis 22:14*

My inspiration for this book's title, *Come Home Alive*, is Louis
Kasischke's account of his 1996 expedition to Mount Everest. Many
people know of the disaster that took place that year when eight climbers
died and several more were stranded. Lou had been a serious mountain
climber for several decades prior to this and knew all the statistics and all
the risks. His enduring love for the mountains and for alpine endurance
sports has taken him to many remote parts of the world, on all seven
continents.[1]

I met Lou at a quality conference in Lansing, Michigan, in 1997
when he was the speaker at one of the breakout sessions. He had us
completely spellbound as he was recounting the quest for the summit
of Everest, six miles up. Lou took us through the physical and mental

1

battle of dealing with your own self. "How will you stay motivated to fight the overwhelming desire to quit?" he asked.

I listened intently to what Lou was sharing with us from his journey. The words that I heard and what I wrote down on paper from Lou's speech were connected to my current emotional state. I wrote down what mattered to me at that time. That was 1997. And now, God had provided me the providence to save those notes from seventeen years ago. All those years, and those notes were still there. Why? Because there were words on those pages I had written down and needed to see, to read, and to contemplate.

- The power to harness your will makes all the difference between life and death.
- Teamwork is critical.
- Teammates are what you will need.
- Climbers know how to trim out the waste and carry just what's necessary.
- You must have the strength to get back down the mountain.
- Listen to the unheard, and see the invisible.

Lou's compelling story is not about the endurance and rigor it required to continue on to the summit. Lou was only four hundred feet from achieving his goal to reach the top of Mount Everest. That was not the greater goal. Goal number one was to come back home. He had promised his wife, Sandy, that whatever overwhelming odds, human circumstances, and adverse conditions there were, he would stay true to the order of the goals. His compelling story is about forfeiting the immense desire to succeed and reach the top in order to channel his will for the greater promise to *come back home.*

On one of the nights that was the darkest and the loneliest for me, I came across those notes. They were on three handwritten pages, and I read them repeatedly. This, I sensed, was the cancer fight. How do you deal with your own self? How will you stay motivated to fight the overwhelming desire to quit when the air gets thin, your strength is gone, and you feel like you are freezing to death from the inside out. This would not be my fight, but it would be for my husband, Chris.

What would that be like for him? And how could I help him? How could I be his teammate?

There are times when only alone, in the deep quiet of the dark of night, we are able to discover the most intimate and haunting truths of our lives. How can I use these and other words to help Chris to *come home alive?*

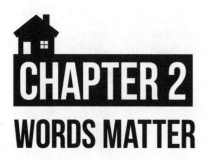

CHAPTER 2
WORDS MATTER

Words, like nature, half reveal and
half conceal the soul within.
—*Alfred Lord Tennyson*

We navigate our whole lives using words. Change and improve
the words and I believe we can change and improve life.
—*Martin Firrell*

My role as a training consultant and communication expert for more than thirty years stretches me to both find and use the right words. I see words, and I say words. I read words, and I write words. I hear words and listen to words. Words are important to me. The words I use are fairly simple. I am not an eloquent speaker or a gifted writer. I just want to say it in a way that all can understand. Not only are the right words important for me to say, but I also know that by listening intently, I can get the message that others intend me to hear. Communication is described as talking and listening. It has two parts. We must do both. For all those years, I have taught people how to develop listening skills. We remember 90 percent of what we teach others. Now was going to be the time when this needed to pay off for me. How can I listen to comprehend the complete message? The psalmist says, "The unfolding of your words gives light; it gives understanding" (Psalm 119:130). The words I needed to hear were everywhere.

- Send angels with armor.
- Lose the weight of it.
- Guard your lips to guard your life.
- "My Presence will go with you and I will give you rest" (Exodus 33:14).
- This type of cancer is in epidemic proportions.
- That will just be the greatest thing.
- You are not a doctor.
- A big life day.
- He is at coma levels; get to the emergency room now.
- Don't pretty it up.
- This could go either way.
- Nothing bad lasts forever.
- My, how you have aged.
- We'll need to do another biopsy.
- There are some troubling symptoms.
- The tumor is growing uncontrollably.
- I will take you to the doorstep of death and bring you back again.
- It's just the fear of the unknown.
- Be stellar.
- Piece of cake.
- Choose the better thing.
- Follow the highlighted route.
- Your tumor is melting like ice off a hot tin roof.
- Make good friends and good choices.
- You are here to bring life and growth to others.
- Listen to the unheard, and see the invisible.
- You're accepted.
- "And now these three remain: faith hope and love. But the greatest of these is love" (1 Corinthians 13:13).

For twenty years, God has been leading, guiding, and preparing me to walk alongside my husband through the diagnosis of throat cancer (2013), the treatment of that cancer (2014), the recovery from all the side effects of the treatments (2015), and then through rehabilitation (2016) to get back to what will be his "new normal" in life. The words I heard and learned over those twenty years were pivotal to playing my role well as his caregiver.

CHAPTER 3
RUNNING RENEGADE

Most of us have enough areas in our lives where we have to meet others' expectations. Let your running be about your own hopes and dreams.
—Meb Keflezighi

The obsession with running is really an obsession with the potential for more and more life.
—George Sheehan

I run. Why do I run? In my running, I seek a sense of peace. I think of it as a clear and sound mind. My mother has questioned my motives over the years. She thinks I am running from something. That is simply not the case. My current motivation to run is because both of my parents lived with heart disease and high blood pressure. My father died of a massive heart attack at the age of sixty-nine. Too young. My mother suffered what we believe was a heart attack as a result of the shock of the situation, was hospitalized in ICU for a week, and was not at my father's funeral. That's why I run.

Running is central to my life because it is a time for me to break away from the pressures of the world and be alone. I don't run with a group. I run *seul*. I am a running renegade. Being alone allows me to change routes on a dime. I can always add on another loop here or there, and I am not weighed down by the structure of the group. It would be a lovely luxury to run with others, but my running time is my praying time, and I need to be alone. This is my most personal alone time, when I can concentrate on the people I care so much about and raise them up to my God and Father for a mile.

We moved in April 2016 from our beloved Central Park neighborhood of fifteen years. One of our mayors called this Central Park neighborhood "Key West without the chickens." It is filled with one-hundred-year-old cottages that border the south side of Lake Macatawa in Holland, Michigan. Many of the houses are small, and the streets are narrow. We know each other. We help each other out. But the neighborhood also includes grand mansions, especially on South Shore Drive. This is where residents with the name Prince, Padnos, DeVos, and Jurries live. I loved the conversion of these two paths—the grand and the modest. The palatial and the subdued. Over the years, I probably had run most of the streets and thoroughfares within eight miles of my home. But in April, we moved to a condominium complex on the complete opposite side of town. Now I will need to find new routes, new houses to connect with, and new streets and sidewalks to learn so I don't misstep and fall.

The neighborhood was different. My new running routes took me through more commercial areas, up against speeding cars on wide lanes of traffic. It just wasn't the same. I wasn't running as much. There was always some kind of excuse. My connection to God seemed severed. My heart felt dead. The harder I tried to like my new streets and paths, the more I resisted them and simply stopped my training routine—until one day when I heard the words "You will be uncomfortable; get over it." The conversation went something like this:

> You have been pretty comfortable for the last fifteen years on your journey. Now I have something bigger I want you to do with your life. I have been pouring many lessons into you for the past twenty years. Use those lessons for My glory.

And so, on August 13, 2016, I prayed:

- What on earth am I here for? (Sound familiar? Yes, I was reading Rick Warren's *Forty Days of Purpose*.)
- Help me to know Your will for my life.
- May this seed that you have put in me take root and bear much fruit.
- What are you wanting to speak to me in the deepest chambers of my heart?

I was also reading John Eldredge's *The Ransomed Heart*. It is a collection of devotional readings from the various books he has authored—*Wild at Heart, The Journey of Desire, The Sacred Romance, Waking the Dead, Captivating, and Epic*.

My August 13 reading was an excerpt from *Waking the Dead*:

> Denial is a favorite method of coping for many Christians. But not with Jesus. He wants truth in the inmost being, and to get it he's got to take us into our inmost being. One way he'll do this is by bringing up an old memory. You'll be driving down the road and suddenly remember something from your childhood … However he brings it up, go with him there. He has something to say to you … These are all invitations to go with him into the deep waters of the heart, uncover the lies buried down there, and bring in the truth that will set us free. Don't just bury it quickly: ask God what he is wanting to speak to.[1]

What are You wanting to speak to me in the deepest waters of my heart? He would reveal the answer a few days later when I was on day seven of *The Purpose Driven Life*:

> God didn't give you your abilities for selfish purposes. They were given to benefit others, just as others were given abilities for your benefit … Jesus stood at a fork in the road. Would he fulfill his purpose and bring glory

to God, or would he shrink back and live a comfortable, self-centered life? You face the same choice.[2]

In 1 Peter 4:10–11 we read:

Each one should use whatever gift he has received to serve others, faithfully administering God's grace in its various forms. If anyone speaks, he should do it as one speaking the very words of God. If anyone serves, he should do it with the strength God provides, so that in all things God may be praised through Jesus Christ. To him be the glory and the power for ever and ever. Amen.

In an instant, I was reminded of some powerful words I heard on mile twenty-five of the 2007 Chicago Marathon: *My child, I love you, and I have mercy on you; I give you my grace, and I give you my guidance; now go and do likewise.* And then the Lord placed Acts 20:24 on my heart: "However, I consider my life worth nothing to me, if only I may finish the race and complete the task the Lord Jesus has given me."

The writing will be difficult and the ultimate message that I will need to share will be profoundly uncomfortable. The next morning, I was out on the road with the realization that this daunting journey begins with a training run today, not tomorrow. I must begin to face my fears on these new paths, roads, and highways. The area we live in is called "the heights." It bears that name for a reason. The hills are grueling. I would need to make the effort to embrace the challenge, muster the energy, and tackle the terrain. How can I make this into my new routine? How can I see these new homes and neighborhoods as my friends? Where, in all this uncomfortableness, can I become more aware of God's glory? This will be uncomfortable.

My favorite musical artist is Simply Red. One of his songs, "For Your Babies," was playing in my ears just as I turned the corner for home that day. My focus will be for the generations yet unborn. "They will proclaim his righteousness to a people yet unborn—for he has done it" (Psalm 22:31).

Toby Mac gets it right with his lyrics in "Speak Life."

> Raise your thoughts a little higher, use your words to
> inspire
>
> Joy will fall like rain when you speak life with the
> things you say.[3]

Understand that I have not always spoken life to others. There have been times when inappropriate words to others and about others came out of my mouth. For those that were on the receiving end, I apologize and ask for your forgiveness.

Today, one in every three females and one in every two males will be diagnosed with cancer in their lifetime. But new statistics show that a child born today—male or female—has a one in two chance of developing cancer at some point in his or her life.[4] A cell will go rogue, and that's how it starts. In 2020, 606,520 people are projected to die of cancer in the United States.[5]

Cancer is one struggle, but there are countless others: relationships that are strained or estranged; bills and bill collectors that will not go away. Cancer is one of the five big killers. The other four are: cardiovascular disease, Alzheimer's disease, diabetes, and pulmonary disease.[6] "People are most receptive to God when they are under tension or in transition," says Rick Warren in his mega best seller *40 Days of Purpose*.[7] In *Moving Mountains*, John Eldredge says,

> If you say that God does not intend to use affliction, then
> what in your mind does he then use? Joy does wonderful
> things for our souls—it soothes, and strengthens, and
> heals. But joy does not transform people's characters in
> the same way affliction does. You do not grow when
> life is good.[8]

If you are in that place, I hope you will be receptive to these words. My prayer is that this book will reach just the right people at just the right time. My prayer is that the words printed here will touch the numb and dying parts of your heart to bring life and growth to you again. My prayer is for renewed energy for all the caregivers in the world and for you to know that what you do every day and night matters. My prayer is that these words in some small way can heal the cancers in your marriage, your relationships, and your work. My prayer is that your fears will subside, and you will experience real peace. My prayer is for full and complete healing and restoration for any who suffer from the diseases in our world.

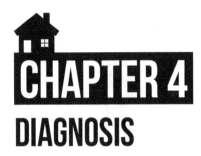

CHAPTER 4

DIAGNOSIS

He who lets the sea lull him into a sense
of security is in very grave danger.
—Hammond Innes

Truth is like the sun. You can shut it out
for a time, but it ain't going away.
—Elvis Presley

The words of Jim Collins from the 2010 Leadership Summit rang in my ears: "When do you know that you are sick on the inside?" He was sharing a story about his wife, Joanne Ernst. She is a former triathlete and won the 1985 Hawaii Ironman. They were together scaling El Capitan in Yosemite Valley, and she was already sick on the inside, and neither knew. Later she was diagnosed with breast cancer.

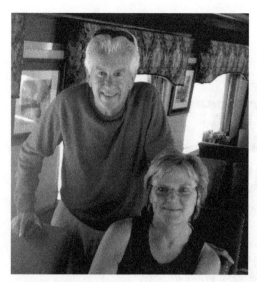

Great Smoky Mountains Vacation August 2013

When do you know you are sick on the inside? Two months before his diagnosis, Chris was extremely sick, and we didn't even know it. After eight months of not feeling well and requesting a second opinion, Chris and I found ourselves stunned, speechless, and physically ill when we heard the diagnosis of throat cancer. He wasn't a smoker and had never used tobacco products. Throat cancer. Wow.

It all started with a request for a second opinion after the original diagnosis of acid reflux. Four months later the ensuing treatment was getting us nowhere, with the symptoms getting worse by the week. He still had a constant sore throat, abnormal weight loss, and little or no energy to get through the day.

Our primary care physician was able to refer us to another ears, nose, and throat doctor. This new specialist was Dr. Richard Strabbing, and without using an instrument of any type, he knew there was a tumor in Chris's neck. "Late stage three, maybe early stage four," as he looked down Chris's throat. The scope confirmed his visual diagnosis that there was some type of abnormal growth in the back of his mouth near his vocal cords. "We will need to prepare for a biopsy immediately." A biopsy is what is necessary to get a sample of the cells or tissue that need examination. During the biopsy, tissue is removed and examined for proper diagnosis of the mass or tumor that is growing abnormally. This would be scheduled for the earliest time on Dr. Strabbing's schedule.

My first encounter with cancer was in 1974 when my father was diagnosed with colon cancer and needed surgery to remove the tumor. I was only twenty at the time, so I may not have understood the stark reality of the diagnosis. Or what this might mean for my father's quality of life, or if he even would live past his late forties.

We were gathered at the hospital—my mother, my two brothers, and me. (My sister, who is a nurse, was unable to be there. But she was providing direction from her home in Texas.) After his surgery, my father's bed was being wheeled back into his hospital room, and he was slowly regaining consciousness from the anesthetic. We had met with the surgeon minutes earlier where we heard a positive yet guarded diagnosis. "We removed twelve inches of your father's colon and removed the malignant mass, but there may be some lymph nodes that could be affected nearby. We don't believe there are any affected lymph nodes, but our course of treatment will include chemotherapy as a precaution." All of us heard the surgeon's words, and I tried to digest them as quickly as I could, because one of us would be sharing this with dad. One of us would have to tell him what we knew he did not want to hear, and to provide the support and encouragement that would be so necessary. My brothers are twins, six years older than me. They are oftentimes on the same page and completing each other's sentences. Immediately I heard, "Got to get back to work." And an echo, "Got to get back to work." Then my mother looked at me and said, "I can't tell him; I can't even go in there." So, the words were up to me. How do you even plan for that?

On the day of Chris's biopsy, no one left me on my own. Dr. Strabbing was straightforward and direct. He was present, and he did all the talking. I had all I could do to keep from vomiting.

The thing I remember most from that day was a reaffirmation by Dr. Strabbing that we are looking at a late stage three or stage four tumor.

For whatever reason everything along the way seemed to be complicated. The months of not feeling well, the unaccounted-for weight loss, the delay in an accurate diagnosis, and now the results of the biopsy were not clear. The original pathology indicated some unspecified squamous cell abnormality but not a malignant cancer. This was good news. This was great compared to what we were prepared to hear. Complete and total despair one day and euphoria the next. But Dr. Strabbing was not convinced. He had seen it, examined it, and believed without a doubt we were dealing with a malignant tumor that needed an immediate course of action.

"I'm going to call in 'the closer' on this one. Do you know Willie Hernandez?" Well, Chris reacted with a powerful yes. There were tears in his eyes and emotion could be heard in this one word. I looked at both of them and said, "Fill me in."

"If I would want to save the game, I'd call in Willie Hernandez," said Dr. Strabbing. Willie Hernandez is a major league baseball relief pitcher who was voted the American League's Most Valuable Player (MVP) in 1984, the year the Detroit Tigers won the World Series. A relief pitcher, or closer, specializes in getting the final outs in a close game when his team is leading. This role is often assigned to the team's best reliever. In 1984 for Detroit, Hernandez was that guy. He had saved thirty-two games in thirty-three opportunities. His only blown save came when Detroit had already secured the AL East Division title.[1] Thirty-two saves in thirty-three opportunities. I liked those odds.

Our closer was Dr. Mark E. P. Prince, professor and division chief, head and neck surgery, Department of Otolaryngology, residency director of the University of Michigan hospital in Ann Arbor. Our next step would be to meet this "closer." But when would that be?

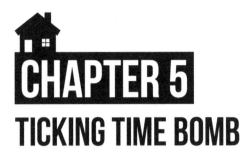

CHAPTER 5
TICKING TIME BOMB

*The mind ought sometimes to be diverted
that it may return to better thinking.*
—*Phaedrus*

*The world is all gates, all opportunities,
strings of tension waiting to be struck.*
—*Ralph Waldo Emerson*

Okay. I'll admit it. I am a *Castle* rerun junkie. During the winter, I can watch three episodes back-to-back-to back on the TNT Channel. I only got wind of the show perhaps in its third season. Probably because I'm generally sleeping before 9:00 p.m. and would never even have the TV on at its normal airing at 10:00 p.m. During one episode, after tracking a killer to his apartment, Beckett steps on a bomb trigger and must stand in place while the bomb squad finds a way to defuse it. Castle stays with Beckett, and they banter back and forth about their relationship over the years. As it's a television show, the complete episode is strewn with flashbacks from previous seasons. The sole purpose: to distract Beckett from the fact that with the slightest movement, everything could blow to smithereens.

Even after Castle was mandated to evacuate the building with ten minutes left on the timer before detonation, he manages to come back in with her favorite coffee beverage and ultimately to crack the code—find the password and eliminate the threat.[1]

A ticking time bomb is a problematic situation that will eventually become dangerous if not addressed. Together, we were a ticking time bomb:

- The reality was the diagnosis of a suspicious growth in his throat.
- The biopsy confirmed the tumor, but the results were unclear and, in fact, inconclusive.
- Our appointment with Dr. Prince was not until November 22.
- We had no clue what the next steps were, or even a time frame on which to base our lives.
- Chris needed a massive distraction.

We headed to Chicago for the weekend where two of our grown sons live. The agenda: take a Segway tour.

We all came from different parts of town, so we met up at the tour office. The exact diagnosis was not final yet, so their reaction and our conversation were interesting. It was almost like nothing is wrong and nothing will be wrong, except everything is wrong and it all will blow up, perhaps momentarily. "The 'easy way' is our laziness trying to find a solution by 'working hard' to side-step the problem," says Craig D. Lounsbrough. We were doing just that.

Chris and I had already been on a Segway tour through downtown Philadelphia several years back. It was the same month, November, and at that time, we were the only ones to sign up. What a luxury to have the leader devote his time exclusively to us, so we could learn how to control our new personal transportation device through the historic sites and statues of downtown Philadelphia. It takes concentration to learn how to drive/ride a Segway. Each slight move you make left or right, forward or backward is a command to be carried out. You will head that way even if the path is not clear. But once you get it, it is a load of fun.

The tour in Chicago on that day had other families just like us. We were potentially seen as "old hats" and even helped some of the newbies.

Keep the distractions coming. Our tour took us through the Grant Park and museum campus area. Buckingham Fountain was pretty deserted, so we could get accustomed to the machine and figure out how fast our individual nerves would let each of us go. We could do spins and turns and feel a sense of freedom. Maybe the bomb wouldn't go off after all, or better yet, maybe there wasn't even a bomb. We were still in shock, and for sure in the denial phase.

We stopped halfway through the tour for some hot chocolate and caught up on "other" things. We simply avoided the ticking time bomb scenario. Our tour then took us over to the museum campus around the Natural History Museum, and then down the long drive to the planetarium. The finale was touring around old Meigs Field and then back to the planetarium periphery for our photo shoot. This was total and complete success in the distraction department. The guide had no clue about the news we'd heard about a week ago. Now, what's the next distraction?

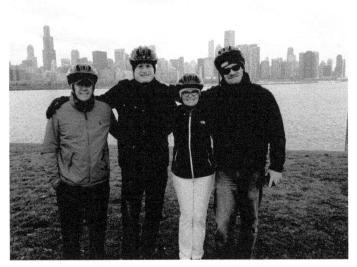

Segway tour of downtown Chicago

CHAPTER 6
LIGHT FOR THE WAY
THEY SHOULD TAKE

Hope is being able to see that there is
light despite all of the darkness.
—Desmond Tutu

Faith is the strength by which a shattered
world shall emerge into the light.
—Helen Keller

What is trust? "Trust is a reliance on, integrity, strength, ability, surety and confidence in a person or a thing."[1] There are many people we trust the most, and we haven't even met them. Airplane pilots come first to mind. You get on an airplane; you buckle your seatbelt. The flight attendant gives the preflight instructions. The plane taxis to the runway. You take off and enjoy your flight. You land and get off the plane, and that's that. You just put your life into the hands of the flight crew, and you probably didn't know any of them. But you trust them with your life.

Many of us are familiar with the story of Chesley Sullenberger, known best as Sully. The movie with Tom Hanks playing the pilot has exposed his heroism of perfectly landing a commercial aircraft with 155 souls on board right in the middle of the Hudson River in New York. When those passengers boarded their flight that morning, they were probably not thinking about the credentials and experience of the captain or the crew. They were probably not focused on all the worst-case scenarios. Or how well equipped each of the crew members were to handle any number of emergency situations. They didn't ask for their business cards or their resumes. They trusted. And boy did Sully deliver with his instantaneous decision making and execution that resulted in every single person on board coming home alive.[2]

Trusting a person implies that we rely on them. We have confidence in their abilities. We have an expectation that in their care, all will be well. Trust implies hope. Things will work out if we just trust. Sarah Young in her *Jesus Calling* devotional says, "Trust is a golden pathway to heaven."[3]

One of our most special vacation spots is Hilton Head Island. Hilton Head is known for its miles of bike paths. We have vacationed there now over ten times. Each time we have stayed, we are in a different timeshare. Some are located near each other, and others are not. During one visit in February we were staying in Sea Pines. The bike trails are numerous. Many of them head to the famous Harbour Town area where the Harbour Town golf course is located. During the daylight on our bikes, it seems so easy, even though the trails are far from straight. They weave in and around this big tree and that obstacle. Every now and then, the signage directs us to cross the street, and then the path picks up on that side of the road for a while. You must pay attention, so you can stay on the designated path—on the correct path, the one you should be on. You will be safe there.

I run in the early morning—most often around 5:00 a.m. The saying goes, "It is darkest before the dawn." And on Hilton Head, remarkably close to the Atlantic Ocean, nothing could be truer. I had the knowledge of seeing the path ahead of time. I saw the numerous switchbacks. I could somewhat get the lay of the land. But without a flashlight, I wouldn't even think of taking that route in the dark.

Twice in the Bible we read of the pillar of cloud and pillar of fire for guidance. Exodus 13:21 says, "By day, the Lord went ahead of them in a pillar of cloud to guide them on their way, and by night in a pillar of fire to give them light, so they could travel by day or night." In Nehemiah 9:12 we read: "By day you led them with a pillar of cloud, and by night with a pillar of fire to give them light on the way they were to take."

When you are on a cancer journey, whether it's day or night, you are feeling your way in the dark. There is uncertainty, fear, desperation, silence, depression, anxiety, fright, and panic. I'm sure there are a whole host of words that I have missed. We need all the help we can get. We need a pillar of cloud by day and a pillar of fire by night. In a cancer fight, we need to cling and grasp on to a trustworthy hand. "For I am the Lord, your God, who takes hold of your right hand and says to you, 'Do not fear; I will help you.'" (Isaiah 41:13).

Leading up to our appointment where we would learn the outcome of the biopsy, I was taking hold of Dr. Prince's hand by going online to review his curriculum vitae, or CV, as many people say. I wanted a quick way to understand the man, his skills, and his qualifications. His credentials were broad and extensive, and this gave me much confidence. While we didn't yet have any definitive answers, we sure felt as if we were surrounded by a team in whom we could put our total and complete trust. While we were waiting, we would hold God's hand in childlike trust. God was sending this earthly doctor as our step-by-step guide to make our path straight. We could trust him. And we hadn't even met him—our closer.

We met Dr. Prince for the first time on November 22, 2013. In Michigan, the place to go for complex diagnosis and care is the University of Michigan Hospitals in Ann Arbor. We were in the right place. He had received the results of the biopsy and the University of Michigan cancer board was to have met prior to our arrival. This is a group of peers that all put their heads together to determine the exact diagnosis and then course of action. Dr. Prince established trust with us right away. He was kind, straightforward, and appeared to have years of experience. Dr. Strabbing wanted him on the team, because if surgery was to be an option, he was the real deal.

Letters and numbers are essential to our everyday living. But they can be terrifying when referred to in the stage of cancer. My sister, the nurse, kept asking, "What stage is it?" There is a standard staging system that acts as a tool for doctors, so they are all on the same page. It is called the TNM system.

In the TNM system, each cancer is assigned a letter or number to describe the tumor, node, and metastases.

- T stands for the original (primary) tumor. Numbers after the T (such as T1, T2, T3, and T4) might describe the tumor size and/ or spread into nearby structures. The higher the T number, the larger the tumor and/or the more it has grown into nearby tissues.
- N stands for nodes. It tells whether the cancer has spread to the nearby lymph nodes. The higher the N number, the greater the spread.
- M stands for metastasis. It tells whether the cancer has spread to distant parts of the body. M0 means there is no evidence of any spread. M1 or M2 would mean that metastasis was found in other organs or tissues.[4]

Our letters and numbers were: T4 N2b M0. Translation: late stage invasive squamous cell carcinoma, with spread to two nearby lymph nodes, but no metastasis. Praise the Lord!

Stage four is the last stage. "The biggest issue with throat cancer is its detection which usually occurs in advanced stages, and this late detection also reduces the effects of the treatment. At this stage, the cancer has already spread to the lymph nodes and other organs. Its further advancement can only be prevented by aggressive treatment, which includes a combination of radiation and chemotherapy sessions with surgery. While the early stages are treatable, prognosis is quite poor in the advanced stages. Survival of the patient usually depends on his/ her health, the effect of the treatment and will-power."[5]

So, Chris's tumor is severe; it has advanced. It is stage four. The tumor is larger and has spread into nearby structures. This is probably why it is so difficult for him to swallow, and even to breathe at times. While this was frightening to hear, at least the full team knew what we were dealing with, and now a plan and time line could be developed for the proper treatment to attack and annihilate this thing.

What is the next step? Many fine doctors at the University of

Michigan, trained in just these situations, put their heads together and determined that given the size, the growth, and the position of the tumor, if surgery were to be performed, it would require a partial pharyngectomy, partial glossectomy, and laryngectomy with neck dissections. In layman's terms, it would be an extensive surgery and would require postsurgical reconstruction. Chris might lose half of his neck. When doing surgery of this type, Dr. Prince indicated there is great concern for "loss of voice, quality of life, and facial disfiguration." Dr. Prince gave us the verdict: "Given the extent of the surgery required, the tumor board feels that chemoradiation therapy would be the most appropriate therapy." So, he was going to get radiation and chemotherapy together—concurrently, at the same time. How will he handle this?

As we walked out the door of his office on November 22, the research student was waiting, ready to pounce. She was standing there with her clipboard filled with a stack of papers. That's what the University of Michigan is about—they do research. But it was just too early. I needed to think through and process what I had just heard. *Really? Now you want us to meet with a young student so Chris can be a part of a massive study?* Yes, we want to help, but the timing of this was bungling, awkward, intrusive, and completely inappropriate. I just needed to get past her to make my way to the bathroom as quickly as I could.

CHAPTER 7
DO NOT BE AFRAID

We are not to be anxious about the unknown future or to fret about it. We are to live in a moment-by-moment dependence upon God.
—James Montgomery Boice

Nothing in life is to be feared. Now is the time to understand more, so that we may fear less.
—Marie Curie

There are many preparations before you can actually start with the treatment. A full PET scan needs to be done, a feeding tube needs to be put into the abdomen, a chemo port needs to be installed, and the mask for his head has to be measured and made so the radiation can be targeted to just the right area in his throat each weekday.

In 1985, we went on a vacation to the Bahamas and met Marvin and Bitty. Marv was an attorney for the City of Dallas, and we met because we were staying at the same hotel. Chris and I loved to snorkel, so we brought our own equipment and found out-of-the-way little beaches to snorkel and look for varieties of fish. We asked Marvin and Bitty to join us one day and use our equipment. We showed them what to do and hoped they would enjoy the experience as much as we did.

Marvin was in the water about two hundred feet out from the

shoreline when we saw him stand up quickly. The water came up to just over his knees. He came walking back to us after only being out for about five minutes. "How was it Marv," Chris asked? "Isn't it beautiful out there? Anything wrong, you're back so soon?" Marvin looked at both of us and, in a soft voice, said, "It's just the fear of the unknown."

That would totally describe our emotions. That's where we found ourselves heading into the final weeks of 2013. Each of us was in unknown waters. They might have only come up to our knees, but for all we knew we were dumped in the middle of the Atlantic Ocean with no life support and Hurricane Matthew[1] coming up on our tails.

Our pastor, Todd VanEk, prayed over us these words from Isaiah: "When you pass through the waters, I will be with you; and when you pass through the rivers, they will not sweep over you. When you walk through the fire, you will not be burned; the flames will not set you ablaze" (Isaiah 43:2). Todd continued, "Something that may be comforting to dwell on when the water overtakes you is to know that God is taking you specifically through these troubled waters because your enemies can't swim."

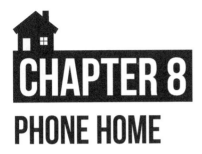

CHAPTER 8
PHONE HOME

When you're safe at home you wish you were
having an adventure; when you're having an
adventure, you wish you were safe at home.
—Thornton Wilder

A man travels the world over in search of what
he needs and returns home to find it.
—George Moore

My homes. Every time I count them, it comes up to eighteen. I've done the recount several times in my head as well as on paper, because I just don't want to forget one. Home. What is home for you? I needed the stability of my childhood home. "Family is the feeling that your HEART is home again," is the caption on a picture frame where I have one of the most precious pictures of my mom, brothers, and sister.

When you are afraid, and unknowns are overtaking you, *phone home*! Even E.T.—the extraterrestrial—knew what was best for him when he was sick.[1] Phone home to your heavenly Father, but go home to your earthly family.

A tradition with us over the years for the Thanksgiving holiday is to drive south to Wilmington, North Carolina, on the Atlantic coast. My brother and sister-in-law have been great hosts to us over the years giving us a warm blast of sea air before heading into the cold and sometimes excessive snow during the winter months along the western coast of Michigan. My mother lives there too, just five minutes from them. A great delight was that at the last minute our son, Ara, could join us for the trip. This provided a safe cocoon of family that is so important when your world is shocked to its core. When I saw my mom, I precisely knew the excitement of E.T.—the extraterrestrial. E.T., phone home; E.T., phone home!

CHAPTER 9
THE GIFT OF PRESENCE

Being present with those who suffer is, in fact, the greatest
gift we can give because it communicates love made flesh.
—Joe E. Pennel Jr.

The meeting of two eternities, the past and the
future ... is precisely the present moment.
—Henry David Thoreau

The hours in the car going home provided an opportunity to read the book *The Gift of Presence*, by Joe E. Pennel Jr. When not driving, this was my distraction from the anxiety of what the next week and month would bring. The book is small and can be read in one sitting. It's a guidebook for professional caregivers and those who find themselves needing to be with and comfort those who are suffering. "We offer those who are suffering a sacred gift when we agree to be present to their pain. Physical presence, silence, and sincerity are of utmost importance as we reach out to those who suffer."[1]

Many of us find ourselves at a loss for just what to say to someone. You don't have to say anything. Just be present. One friend and his sons came by one afternoon to shovel the snow off our roof. Another friend came by to bring muffin dough. I could decide the number of muffins I wanted to bake at one time, on my own. It was perfect. Not many words were said with each of these visits, but those gestures will last forever.

You will need to talk at some point. Your words matter. So, choose them wisely. Share words that provide a sense of hope. Pennel says, "There is a disease more devastating than suffering. It is hopelessness." During one of Chris's hospital stays a nutritionist came in to get some details. She asked Chris where he lived. I was standing next to him, and so he said, "I live with her." She assumed I was Chris's daughter. Yes, his facial features were not the same as before he became ill, he had lost fifty pounds, and indeed he looked frail. She came up to me afterward to apologize and express her regret for saying what she had. She acknowledged this was a good lesson for her, and she should have known better as she talks with and provides nutritional advice to cancer patients all the time. When visiting and sharing your gift of presence, take care and be sensitive to someone's appearance that has changed because of the disease and the treatment plan. Don't let your natural sense of perception rule your tongue. I heard someone say to a cancer patient, "you look twenty years older since I saw you last." The thought may be there, and the appearance may be real, but tick a lock. Button it up.

A special passage I kept near to my heart was, "Guard your lips to guard your life." It is based on Proverbs 13:3. I reviewed many Bible translations but found the Contemporary English Version to land the dismount for me, "Keep what you know to yourself, and you will be safe; talk too much and you are done for." I learned to react slowly to sensitive words that I heard. I tried to get past specific words that were hurtful and focus on giving people the benefit of the doubt. One time I heard the inference that if I gave my husband more sex at this time he'd bounce back to life. I am glad the individual came to me personally to apologize for those words spoken in jest and in haste. It is important to think about how the words will come out and how they will be interpreted. It is great to put a smile on someone's face, but think through the joke first. What's even better, don't tell it.

We have all experienced words that upended us, buckled us, bent us over, trapped us, stopped us, and demoralized us. A wise tongue can bring healing. When I pondered this passage, "Reckless words pierce like a sword, but the tongue of the wise brings healing" (Proverbs 12:18), I realized this is a promise we can cling to. Our words do bring healing. We can heal others. God will honor that promise with our words.

My sister-in-law, Donna, is my prayer warrior. She always has the right words and the right prayers, and she just never gives up. Her words bring healing to me. She was my texting partner from the moment that the diagnosis was confirmed. Through her texting, she was virtually present. Even though I was alone, I felt together with her.[2] That gave me peace.

The Seven Simple Do's and Don'ts from *The Gift of Presence* are gems for those of us who are spouses, relatives, friends, and professional caregivers:

1. Be a good listener. Let your words be few (Ecclesiastes 5:2). Try to listen beyond signs, words, and sounds to really hear what is going on in the depths of the person's soul.
2. Do not say, "I know how you feel." It is better to say, "Tell me how you are feeling."
3. Do not be a busybody. Receive what the sufferer is willing to share at that time.
4. Do not overstay your visit.
5. Avoid using rote sayings.
6. Offer practical help.
7. Listen to the stories.[3]

We were at the beginning of December, and the treatments would not start until after the New Year. We were meeting with our lawyer, Nathan Bocks, at this time, and he reassured us confidently. Their son, Duncan, was diagnosed with acute lymphocytic leukemia (ALL) at twenty months, and they began treatments *immediately*. "This is good. This is good. Look at it this way," he said, "you'd be in there right now if it was life threatening. With Duncan we went straight from diagnosis into treatment."

The Gospels list about 125 statements Christ made. Of those, twenty-one urge us to "not be afraid" or "not fear" or "have courage" or "take heart" or "be of good cheer." If quantity is any indicator, Jesus takes our fears seriously. The one statement He made more than any other was this: Do not be afraid. Do whatever it takes to keep your eyes on Jesus. When you are afraid—pray. On our list of fears, the fear of what's next demands a prominent position. When the fear of what's next comes upon you, remember what Jesus said, "I will ask the Father, and he will give you another Counselor to be with you forever" (John 14:16). The Holy Spirit—counselor, friend, helper, intercessor, advocate, strengthener, standby.[4]

> If you feel like you're in a dark place in your circumstances right now, know that God has not abandoned you. He is there with you in great power and wants you to realize how much He loves you. If you're in darkness as a result of your own choices, confess that to Him and He will lead you out of it. If it is a darkness He has created to grow your faith, be joyful. There are awesome treasures of His presence ahead for you.[5]

> Who walks in darkness and has no light? Let him trust in the name of the Lord and rely upon his God. (Isaiah 50:10)

Our plan, rooted in faith and hope, started with daily prayer time together and belief in the healing power of God and in our home team of physicians; and ended with thankfulness and expecting a miracle! What we did together in the middle is one you can do too—through greater awareness of each other's strengths and how to work together and be a team.

This six-point plan was our north star to get through the toughest days and nights:

- Pray.
- Believe.
- Know the patient.
- Know the caregiver.
- Give thanks and be grateful.
- Expect a miracle.

In the same way, the Spirit helps us in our weakness. We do not know what we ought to pray for, but the Spirit himself intercedes for us with groans that words cannot express.

Romans 8:26

PART 2

PRAYER

CHAPTER 10
PRAYER

When I pray, coincidences happen, when I don't, they don't.
—*Archbishop William Temple*

*We can be tired, weary and emotionally distraught, but
after spending time alone with God, we find that He
injects into our battles energy, power and strength.*
—*Charles Stanley*

In 1996, a crisis came into our lives that only prayer could cover. Everything was disrupted in that year. The Lord moved us in such a powerful way to leave one worshipping body and move to another one. Each Sunday, the message, the choir, the hymns, and the dramas all seemed to be just what I needed to touch my broken and crumbling heart. On one Sunday, Ross Nykamp was giving a personal testimony about taking the time to write a love letter to the Lord each day. I have known Ross for many years, as he was on staff at our local Chamber of Commerce, and we worked together on a program called SiBus: Students in Business. That morning, Ross shared how his friend, Mike Bailey, prayed for his children. He prayed specifically for angels with armor to surround Ross's children. Isn't that a beautiful word picture!

I went home from that experience feeling very ashamed for not praying diligently for my own children and thought how important it would be that I start praying for angels with armor to surround my own two sons.

Our youngest son, Geoff, had just recently chosen his life path. He was headed to the University of Michigan on a Naval ROTC scholarship. He didn't know his exact passion and Navy community yet, but knowing that he would be serving our country and placing his life at risk triggered an immediate reaction. I would need to begin fervently praying for Geoff. I prayed, *Dear Lord, send angels with armor to surround him at all times and at all places. Put a capsule of protection around his mind, his heart, and his life.* A few months later the Lord would show me visible proof that He heard those prayers and answered them.

It was the end of April in 1997 and the last day of Geoff's freshman year. Chris and I headed over to Ann Arbor in two cars to pick up Geoff and bring all his belongings back to Holland. My car was a Pontiac Grand Am, a cute, purple, sporty little thing. Geoff would drive that home. I wanted to sit with him in the front seat, but it was needed as a space to load more stuff, so I decided against that and rode back with Chris. We stopped at Chili's in Brighton and even had a Bloomin Onion appetizer. The things we remember. We passed through Lansing headed west on I-96 and right at exit 84, Chris looked in the rearview mirror and said, "Geoff is having an accident."

I turned around quickly to look out of the rear window and saw my son lose control of the car on the right shoulder of Interstate 96, then overcompensate and sail the car across the two lanes of the highway airborne into the median. The car began its roll, crashing to the ground halfway between the lanes of traffic.

As Chris and I looked for a turnaround, I watched as the car landed on all four wheels but was turned 180 degrees with the rear of the car now headed for the opposite two lanes of the eastbound traffic. The car finally lost momentum and came to a stop about two feet from the oncoming traffic.

As we were driving up, I saw all six feet two and 205 pounds of Geoff emerge from the car and stand up! There were no explanations. He simply did not know what had happened. What we saw in the driver's seat was like a capsule. Everything that was packed inside the car was in complete disarray, but where he sat was protected with what appeared to be a capsule of armor. The passenger side and the rear seat were damaged, crashed, and caved in. The car was a total loss.

An ambulance came and took Geoff to the Lansing hospital just to be sure there were no broken bones or internal damages. Finally, when he was all settled in, I went to the bathroom. I got inside this very sterile hospital bathroom and immediately lay down face first on the hard, cold tile floor with my body shaking, totally spread out to the four corners, to thank the Lord for the life of my child. I have never felt so much the presence of the Lord as in that place, and at that time.

Geoff will remember three things about the accident—"Oh no, I'm going to die," "I am now dead," and then, "Why am I not dead?" These are the only things he remembers during those few seconds when the car was airborne and rolling in the median.

There are two tragedies in the world. One is that we have the capacity to help others out and don't. The second and bigger tragedy is when we don't reach out and ask for help. When you are going through the dark night of your soul, reach out and ask for angels with armor to surround you at all times and at all places. When you reach out and ask for help, the help you need will be there.

It was at this time that I discovered I had the spiritual gift of intercession. The gift of intercession is the divine enablement to consistently pray on behalf of and for others, seeing frequent and specific results. I identified this through a tool called Network,[1] which helps you recognize your spiritual gifts.

Intercessors feel compelled to earnestly pray on behalf of someone or some cause. We are convinced that God moves in direct response to our prayers. We are convinced there is real power in prayer. We pray for the protection of others. We are able to carry others' burdens.[2] I am very grateful for this spiritual gift.

I see now that the Lord was asking me to hone, develop, and build that skill. It would take many years of practice crying out on my knees in desperation to be ready for what lay ahead.

I had a great need each day to pray for Chris. We started a prayer ritual, "for where two or three gather in my name, there am I with them" (Matthew 18:20).

The diagnosis, the upcoming treatment, my workload, and the complete stress of it all had me craving for peace. We claimed Exodus 33:14 as our guidepost, and we prayed this with each other daily: "My Presence will go with you and I will give you rest." I could sense and feel this prayer was answered throughout our journey, each and every day. A sermon I heard years ago reverberated in my head. Imagine a preacher unafraid to belt out this message: "I believe, and I will keep on believing in the incredible power of prayer."

This was first and foremost with us each day. Our prayer time included the daily *Jesus Calling,*[3] a daily *Jesus Today*[4] reading, and Peter Scazzero's *Daily Office.*[5] Others that also got into the mix were *The Power of a Praying Life*, by Stormie Omartian,[6] and the daily devotions from the *Couples' Devotional Bible NIV.*[7] We held hands. Some days the tears welled up in our eyes; some days the tears rolled down our cheeks and onto the pages, and some days our crying was in heaves and sobs. But we could truly feel the Presence of the Holy Spirit in the room with us, by us, in us, and through us.

We were not afraid to tell others of Chris's diagnosis. After reading Tom Brokow's *A Lucky Life Interrupted*—the story about his experience with cancer—some reporter was ready to "leak" the story and wanted confirmation of his current health status.[8] We wanted others to know immediately, because we craved their prayers.

During the time of Chris's diagnosis, we were working with the full staff of the Reformed Church in America, as well as the full staff of Faith Reformed Church in Dyer, Indiana. This was certainly no coincidence. God was powerfully at work. Chris and I have worked together since 1995 and often go to these engagements together. A segment of our work involves faith-based nonprofits and churches.

At Faith Church that day, Chris was not feeling well. He looked sick and had lost about fifteen pounds already. What do you do when you are around ministers? You ask them to minister to you. We were all together in their Well Spring gathering place, close to one hundred strong. With arms extended, and as many hands as possible locked on his shoulders and on his head, our friend and pastor, Mike Pitsenberger, asked for total and complete healing of Chris's body, mind, and soul.

Praying for others out loud in their presence becomes a concrete expression of our care and concern for them. I shy away from saying, "I'll pray for you about that." Instead, I want to be with them, to hold hands and be an active partner around concerns that are weighing them down. You can pray whatever comes to mind and whatever is on your heart, or you can come with something more formal and written down.

"Prayer brings a fountain of help that is deeper than the waters of modern medicine or psychology," states Joe Pennel.[9] Prayer has a mysterious power to still the mind, quiet the heart, and minimize stress and anxiety when we are in difficult health, financial, and relationship issues. If you think about it, health, finances, and relationships are the big three issues we deal with in life. There is no doubt. When we were dealing with Chris's cancer diagnosis, I prayed that the Lord would keep the other two—finances and relationship issues—at bay. That prayer was answered.

When praying for the sick and suffering, we need to praise God for the remarkable agents of healing already designed into their bodies. A beautiful prayer for the sick is to ask for God's special grace to use those healing resources to their fullest advantage.[10]

We must never forget that the purpose of prayer is to come into the full knowledge of the will of God. If you want to know the will of God, then read the Bible. I like this thought: Bible = Basic Information Before Leaving Earth. "God desires for us to ask Him about His will for our lives so we can rightfully receive it. We do not want anything to stop His will from being perfectly carried out. I can think of no greater gift than for God to reveal the knowledge of His will—the Bible—to me."[11] When we pray, we must remember that God loves us, has plans for us, and will lay His heart over our hearts as we pray.

Why don't more people pray and pray fervently? I would guess that some people just believe they are wasting their time asking for something that will never occur. Others may see it as an escape route, a way to avoid handling and addressing problems head-on, or to avoid the cold, hard reality of the situation. He has cancer; he is going to die. Pray? What a waste of time.

Some may not pray because they don't believe there is a God. "The Reb," from Mitch Albom's *have a little faith*, uses his years of wisdom and shepherding people in the Jewish faith to wake us up to a different notion. "Oh yes. It is far more comforting to think God listened and said no, than to think that nobody's out there."[12] I believe that God is out there, and He wants to hear my prayers.

There may certainly be times when we think God says no, but maybe He is just saying "not now." Sometimes God does not listen to our prayers because we have disobeyed. Like Jonah, we have gone to Tarshish, instead of where God directed, Nineveh. The story goes like this: Jonah set sail for Tarshish "sailing across the Mediterranean, but not far out, the Lord sent a great wind, so that the ship was nearly broken up in the tempest. The sailors cried out to their individual gods. They woke Jonah and said 'Arise, call on your God; perhaps your God will consider us, so that we may not perish'" (Jonah 1:6 NKJV). But Jonah had a problem. God was not listening to his prayers because he had stubbornly disobeyed Him.[13] If you will confess your sin immediately and ask for forgiveness, God will hear. The lives of your loved ones depend on your confession. Don't wait. Start with God. He has been waiting to hear from you.

"We do not pray to tell God what he does not know, nor to remind him of things he has forgotten. He already cares for the things we pray about … He has simply been waiting for us to care about them with Him."[14] God has been waiting for us to care about what matters to Him. We pray because God likes to be asked. "Prayer is not for the purpose of getting God to help us … but for getting us in line with what God is about to do. Prayer is God's invitation to enter His throne room so He can lay *His Agenda* over our hearts."[15]

Max Lucado says, "Our prayers may be awkward. Our attempts may be feeble. But since the power of prayer is in the One who hears it and not in the one who says it, our prayers do make a difference."[16] Know that your prayers will make a difference.

We must have a submissive heart when we pray. God wants us to be helpless. "Asking for help lies at the root of prayer."[17]

A regular time of prayer, especially in the morning hours, prepares your heart and makes you sensitive to the ways and things of God. God knows what your day holds, and He'll instruct you before you face difficult situations.

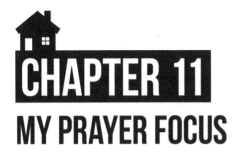

CHAPTER 11

MY PRAYER FOCUS

Praying without fervency is like hunting with a dead dog.
—*Charles Spurgeon*

*Prayer is exhaling the spirit of man and
inhaling the spirit of God.*
—*Edwin Keith*

"My Presence will go with you and I will give you rest" (Exodus 33:14). This became my focus:

- Go straight to God with all your concerns—no matter the time of day.
- Tell it like it is; don't pretty it up.
- Cry out from the bottom of your heart.
- Live believing and expecting answers to your prayers.
- Give thanks for answers that are already under way, even though you haven't seen any outward, visible signs.
- Believe that God's presence is with you, and He desires peace and rest for you as you go about your day.
- Quiet your heart so you don't live in a constant state of tension.
- Praise God and give thanks.

At the close of my prayers, I simply say, "I commend all for whom I pray into your loving arms, trusting and believing that You will answer my prayers according to Your time and according to Your will." Not my time and my will, but according to Your time and according to Your will. This gives me peace to know that God hears me. I am convicted that my God is out there.

> When you look at the life of Jesus you see an absolute trust and confidence that His prayers were not only heard but answered.[1]

"Before a word is on my tongue you, Lord, know it completely" (Psalms 139:4). Jesus teaches us that our basic needs are not met of our own accord, but as a gift from God. Jesus lived this example that times of distress are best handled when we bring others around us to help in carrying the burden. Why did He ask the disciples to come with Him to Gethsemane? He needed them to help Him. But they fell asleep. Prayer is a distinct discipline. It is easy to fall asleep. We need to learn the discipline of prayer so that when the hard and difficult times come, we will be prepared to stay alert, we will be able to hear the will of God, and we will joyfully make intercession for others, because we trust and believe our prayers will be heard and answered. Be someone else's hero today. Pray for them. Remember that everyone, and I mean everyone, is carrying a burden of some sort.

> Prayer releases our lives to the Father and gives Him unhindered access to use us to accomplish His will.[2]

"He is a rewarder of them that diligently seek Him" (Hebrews 11:6 KJV). When you are frightened for your life, say, "I am in trouble, Lord. Help me" (Isaiah 38:14 NLT). This was King Hezekiah's prayer when he became deathly sick. There are times when we are so frightened that this is all we can say. Just earlier he had said more eloquently, "in the prime of my life, must I now enter the place of the dead? Am I to be robbed of the rest of my years?" (Isaiah 38:10–11 NLT).

"The real value of persistent prayer is not so much that we get what we want as that we become the person we should be."[3] I was changing, and Chris was changing. Our prayers were building the belief in us that, in fact, God was listening. Why? We felt an enormous sense of peace. Even if our prayers that Chris would be healed and would live were not immediately visible, just through the act of praying alone, the very Presence of God came to live more fully inside each of us.

My sister-in-law, Donna, was my biggest prayer warrior. "Let us then approach God's throne of grace with confidence, so that we may receive mercy and find grace to help us in our time of need" (Hebrews 4:16). Donna would text me, "I am approaching the throne."

> A tenacious endurance is often the key to victory in prayer. Victory goes to the persistent, not to the angry; to the dedicated, not to those who can provide great demonstrations of emotion and energy. We need committed, determined, systematic prayer, not once in a while fireworks.[4]

As we trust God for all the provisions in our lives, He promises to "make our paths straight" (Proverbs 3:6). The word picture Solomon is giving in this Proverbs verse refers to the ancient practice of highway building. They cleared obstacles, filled in gaps, leveled hills, and cut straight pathways into the sides of mountains. Making our paths straight figuratively means "to facilitate progress" or "turn plans into reality."[5]

As we trust in God and deepen our personal and experiential knowledge of Him, He will facilitate our progress through life and help us successfully follow the path He has marked out for each of us.

> In all your ways submit to him, and He will make your paths straight. (Proverbs 3:6)

> I instruct you in the way of wisdom and lead you along straight paths. (Proverbs 4:11)

It was with that backdrop, coupled with the many books I had read on prayer, and our specific experiences of answered prayer again and again, that we headed into 2014 with a solid foundation upon which we knew God. We were trying to understand His will for our lives. We had faith, trust, and belief that He would answer our prayers in His time and in His way. Don't pray with once-in-a-while fireworks—pray boldly, confidently, and on your knees. God is moved by your prayers.

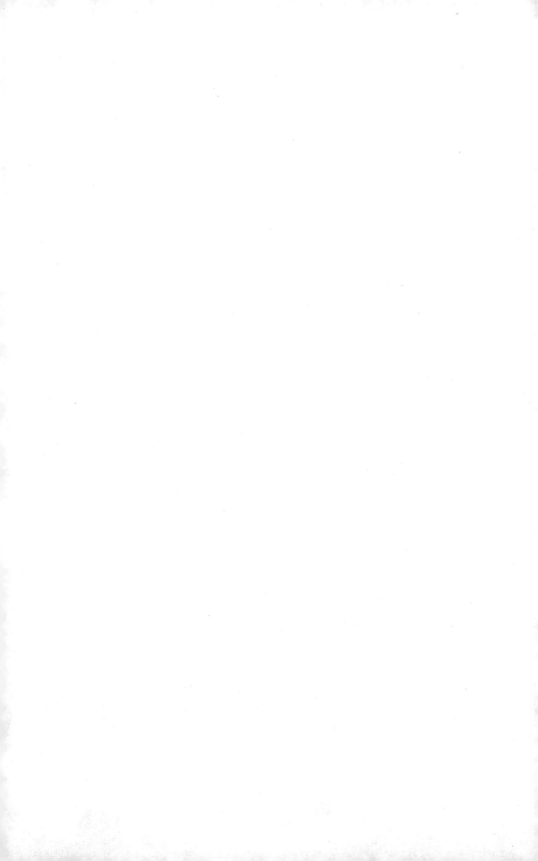

Therefore I tell you, whatever
you ask for in prayer, believe
that you have received it,
and it will be yours.

Mark 11:24

PART 3
BELIEVE

CHAPTER 12

WE BELIEVE

Faith is to believe what you do not see; the reward
of this faith is to see what you believe.
—*Saint Augustine*

Teach me, O God, not to torture myself, not to make
a martyr out of myself through stifling reflection,
but rather teach me to breathe deeply in faith.
—*Søren Kierkegaard*

"Lord, give me the faith to believe, and the patience to hope for answers to my prayers," I would say throughout the day. "Pray, but keep rowing ashore," as a fellow board member used to say when times were tough, and there were more bills than funds to cover them. We need to pray, but we also must take action. Faith is an action. It is a partnership. "One who works in close partnership with God grows in the ability to discern what God wants to accomplish on earth, and prays accordingly," states Philip Yancey.[1]

There is a football coach now at the University of Minnesota by the name of P. J. Fleck. While he was still at Western Michigan University as the head coach during the 2016 season, he was at the center of a Cinderella story. They were undefeated in regular season play. People were drawn to his energy and enthusiasm. He is now attracting talent to play for the Minnesota Gophers away from more traditional football names. Why? Because they believe in him and in his vision. His philosophy starts with three simple words: Row the boat.[2]

Rowing the boat starts with getting the team together in the boat. When everyone is in, they have to be really in. Each person is given two oars, and the practice of working together begins. If you have everyone in the boat rowing at the same pace and in the same direction, the boat will maximize its speed and stay straight. Each person must do his or her part. It's not what each can do individually but what they can do as a team. If someone doesn't row, doesn't keep up, or rows too fast, the boat will zig and zag, or end up going in circles. Energy will be wasted. Everyone must be rowing in harmony to keep the boat straight and headed toward the target.

Row: The R stands for responsibility. Responsibility means being answerable or accountable for something within one's own power, control, or management. Being accountable, that's responsibility.

The: The T stands for trust. Every relationship is built on trust. Developing trust is like constructing a building. It takes time, and it must be done one piece at a time. Trust does not happen without work or effort. Trust results from efforts accumulated over time.

Boat: The B stands for Belief. Rowing a boat is in fact an act of faith. Each one rowing is facing the opposite direction to where the boat is going. We don't know what is ahead of us. All we know is what we have already experienced. You may not know what is coming next, but you can direct your full efforts by one three- or four-second play. Approach the uncertainty one play at a time. Belief is also confidence.[3]

Early on we made a commitment to have total and complete belief in our local system—our local doctors, their expertise, their recommendations … and oh yes, our closer. We felt confident that all the doctors and experts in the boat were in it all the way, and were making their best efforts on our behalf. We just felt this is where God wanted us to be.

Years ago, Chris quit a job that took him on the road each day. On Friday nights, he might be driving back from Indiana, and he was already exhausted from the toll of travel. We needed him to concentrate all the energy he could muster to focus on getting through each three- or four-second play at a time. I didn't want to add commuting, lodging, and navigating that terrain, along with the expense of it, onto his already weary state. He needed to be in a place of consistency, routine, constancy, and safety. He needed to be home.

Our home team consisted of Drs. Strabbing, Hulst, Edlund, and Gribben.

Dr. Strabbing was the doctor who looked at Chris when he walked into the office and knew there was a tumor of some kind already playing havoc on his health. He knew without a doubt that Chris was already sick on the inside. He is an otolaryngologist head and neck surgeon who was born and raised in West Michigan. He is actively involved with teaching medical students.

Dr. Hulst has been Chris's primary care physician for years. He has a special kind of humor and a passion for Corvettes. He started the Lakeshore Corvette Club in Holland, and since Chris has had two Corvettes over his lifetime, there was an instant bond. Dr. Hulst would be the go-to physician for anything outside of the cancer treatments. He and his practice would be the primary contact for anything diabetes-related and keeping Chris's blood sugar levels under control.

Dr. Edlund was his radiation oncologist practicing out of the LAROC facility in Holland. He was our sage, with fifty-four years of experience. He was Chris's encourager who spoke directly to Chris whenever we were meeting with him to share not only his concerns about the progress of the treatment, but also the breakthroughs he was seeing occur since the last visit. He was connected, he was concerned, and he spoke life.

Dr. Gribben was the founding medical director of the St. Mary's Lack's Cancer Center, where he developed an integrated cancer treatment program. The Lack's Center is a state-of-the-art facility that employs a centralized, patient-focused, team approach for improving efficiency and quality of care. We were blessed to have him be our hematologist practicing out of the Cancer and Hematology Center office right in Holland.

"Who among you fears the Lord and obeys the word of his servant? Let the one who walks in the dark who has no light, trust in the name of the Lord and rely upon their God." (Isaiah 50:10). We were walking in the dark, and these were the hands we would hold on to; these were the footsteps we would follow; these were the lights that lead our way. We were certain that God had led them to us, and in them we put our total and complete trust.

> When you are tempted to become fearful, frustrated, uncertain, or panicked about what is happening in your life, stop and see that God is in it. And with Him, you have everything you need for this moment. He knows where you are supposed to be going. And He knows how to get you there.[4]

How do we live with the mystery of unanswered prayer? We must believe. Believe and keep on believing in the incredible, wonderful power of prayer. And then we must wait.

> Once more he visited Cana in Galilee, where he had turned the water into wine. And there was a certain royal official whose son lay sick at Capernaum. When this man heard that Jesus had arrived in Galilee from Judea, he went to him and begged him to come and heal his son, who was close to death. "Unless you people see signs and wonders," Jesus told him, "you will never believe." The royal official said, "Sir, come down before my child dies." "Go," Jesus replied, "your son will live." The man took Jesus at his word and departed. (John 4:46–50)

Jesus didn't wish to travel to Capernaum at that time, and there wasn't a need that He do so. He simply said, "You may go. Your son will live."

> The man took Jesus at his word and departed. While he was still on the way, his servants met him with the news that his boy was living. When he inquired as to the time when his son got better, they said to him, "Yesterday, at one in the afternoon, the fever left him." Then the father realized that this was the exact time at

which Jesus had said to him, "Your son will live." So,
he and his whole household believed. (John 4:50–53)

And then there is the story of the faith of the centurion. A centurion is a professional officer in the Roman Army. In ancient Rome, at the time of Jesus, a centurion was captain over one hundred foot soldiers. A centurion was loyal and courageous, beginning as a soldier in the army and working his way up the ranks. Centurions were noticed by the general for their skill in battle and were made officers. They received pay that amounted to more than twenty times the ordinary soldier's pay.[5]

There was a centurion in Capernaum whose servant was near death. He had heard that Jesus had come back to Capernaum, and being responsible for crowd control, he had often watched Jesus surrounded by large crowds, performing astonishing healing miracles. So, he knew that Jesus could heal.

He was not far from the house when the centurion sent
friends to say to him: "Lord don't trouble yourself, for I
do not deserve to have you come under my roof. That
is why I did not even consider myself worthy to come
to you. But say the word, and my servant will be healed.
For I myself am a man under authority, with soldiers
under me. I tell this one, 'Go,' and he goes; and that one,
'Come,' and he comes. I say to my servant, 'Do this,' and
he does it." When Jesus heard this, he was amazed at
him, and turning to the crowd following him, he said, "I
tell you, I have not found such great faith even in Israel."
Then the men who had been sent returned to the house
and found the servant well. (Luke 7:6–10)

"The centurion had great faith, but this faith was built on practical everyday experience. He already knew that Jesus had healing power. So, he took the principle of obedience in a military chain of command and applied it. He didn't need to be present to ensure that *his* orders were carried out, so logically, neither did Jesus. Like him, Jesus needed only to say the word and it was done," concludes Ed Strauss.[6] What faith this is. What total and complete belief.

All you fathers out there with little daughters can relate to the ruler Jairus. His little girl was dying. Jesus had come to his town. He believed that Jesus was the answer, and so he went to find Him right away. At this time, Jesus had attracted large crowds, and Jairus had his work cut out for him. He needed to push through the multitude of people and get Jesus's attention. He believed if he did that, his daughter would be healed. But he had great respect too, and so upon reaching Jesus, he bowed at His feet and begged, "My little daughter lies at the point of death. Come and lay Your hands on her, that she may be healed, and she will live" (Mark 5:23 NKJV). But some men from his home came to inform Jairus that his daughter was already dead and that Jesus shouldn't be bothered. After hearing news that your daughter is dead and it's essentially over, can you imagine Jesus looking you right in the eye and saying, "Do not be afraid; only believe" (Mark 5:36 NKJV).

"Jairus petitioned Jesus twice—first when his daughter was dying and barely alive, and again after she had just died. He expressed faith in both prayers and never stopped believing that Jesus could heal his daughter. Many people pray and trust God to act in difficult situations, but their faith fails when worse news comes and things suddenly look impossible ... Some people think that when things get desperate, to *continue* praying is bothering the Lord for no reason. But God can not only do the difficult, He can do the impossible," says Ed Strauss.[7]

These are several examples of belief then healing. Belief ... healing. They include others having the faith and belief and pleading on our behalf. These are examples of others' faith. But what about our own faith? Ask the Lord to help you believe beyond your capacity to see the physical evidence of healing right now. We must be bold and confident to seek after God's healing touch. Believe that God can make you whole with just one word or just one touch.

At the same time that Jesus was being called to Jairus's house, a woman with a bleeding problem for twelve years pushed through the crowds and came up behind Jesus to just touch His cloak. "She had suffered a great deal under the care of many doctors and had spent all she had, yet instead of getting better she grew worse." (Mark 5:26)

"If I just touch his clothes, I will be healed. Immediately her bleeding stopped and she felt in her body that she was freed from her suffering" (Mark 5:28–29). "This nameless woman had prayed a silent prayer. She didn't even speak her request. She only thought it. But she had faith in her heart, and when she made contact with Jesus, healing power flowed out of Him into her body. Christians today also need to touch Jesus, to make faith-filled contact with Him," states Ed Strauss in *The Top 100 Prayers of the Bible*.[8]

Boom ... Boom ... Boom. Right after Jairus's daughter and the woman who touched His cloak, two blind men followed him right into Peter's home. How bold! "Jesus asked them, 'Do you believe I can make you see?' 'Yes, Lord,' they told him, 'we do.' Then he touched their eyes and said, 'Because of your faith, it will happen'" (Matthew 9:28–29 NLT). Then they received their sight.

The NLT has Jesus saying, "Because of your faith, it will happen." But in the NKJV, which is closer to the original Greek, He says, "According to your faith let it be to you." This puts the responsibility on us. We must have faith. We will receive answers to our prayers in direct proportion to our faith.

Ed Strauss says, "If you lack faith that God can answer your prayer, soak yourself in His Word and pray for Him to increase your faith. He will do it."[9]

Even the apostles needed to increase their faith. They said this simple prayer, "Lord, increase our faith!" (Luke 17:5) Here is an easy prayer to use if you need help asking for faith during times of duress, distress, disappointment, and disease:

Dear God,

Thank You for Your love for me. Thank You that you accept me. Thank You that I am valuable to You. But I have lost my strength, and I need Your help to increase my faith to believe You will heal my mind, my soul, and my body. I ask that You would strengthen my faith. Increase my faith and strengthen me to move the mountains that block my body from being healed. Help me to keep my faith in You despite my circumstances. Help me to trust that You will never leave me or forsake me. Let me know that You are with me now when I have lost my strength. I pray now in Jesus's name, and I believe You will answer my prayer. Amen.

CHAPTER 13

YOU ARE NOT A DOCTOR

With an awakened heart, we turn and face the
road ahead, knowing that no one can take the
trip for us, nor can anyone plan our way.
—John Eldredge

Whenever you are asked if you can do a job, tell 'em,
"Certainly I can!" Then get busy and find out how to do it.
—Theodore Roosevelt

You are not a doctor. Those words were as clear as if someone was standing right next to me, only the volume was so loud the words had to be coming through the loudspeakers, just above. I had just come to a rest stop during that morning's run right in front of JPs Coffee Shop (now Ferris) on Eighth Street in our downtown.

The loudspeakers are installed in our downtown, as Holland is well known for its annual Tulip Time festival which attracts half a million people during the first two weeks each May. During that time, Eighth Street is abuzz with activities—Klompen dances scheduled nightly, an entourage of geedunk trucks with selections from candy apples to tamales and elephant ears, and lots of parades, each with its own announcer's voices coming through those very speakers. But it was not May; this was February.

Yes, you heard me. You are not a doctor. I bent over at the waist and put my hands on my knees, let out a giant breath through my mouth, and shook and wept uncontrollably. Thank goodness no people were running through the downtown that morning. Normally it is full of an assortment of both runners and walkers due to the snowmelt system in place that keeps all the streets and sidewalks clear of snow and ice. If there had been, they might have crossed to the other side of the street to avoid the crazy lady in front of JPs.

During that month, in the evenings after work, I was on total alert with Chris. Most of the time he was either sitting or sleeping in his chair. He was starting to show signs of weariness through the first seven weeks of treatment. He had weathered them very well, I thought, and even posted a picture of himself on Facebook getting his chemo treatment one Wednesday. He had completed seven chemo treatments and thirty-five radiation treatments with only four radiations to go next week. He was coming down the back stretch with the finish line well in view. So I thought.

The last few days had been rugged for Chris. He probably thought I didn't notice, but his overall energy had changed dramatically. He was sleeping mostly, he said, and trying to force himself to maintain his feedings.

My work demands were so intense for a February. I was working with several teams from the Nestlé division of Gerber Foods in Fremont. The winter was bitterly cold and the hour and a half drive to and from Fremont had me battling snow and treacherous roads. I had been on the road virtually every day by 6:00 a.m. for the past two weeks.

That Friday night was difficult. I heard him get out of bed and leave the bedroom, but the "thud" woke me up and onto my feet in a hurry. He was down on the floor. I hurried over to him, but he didn't move at all or acknowledge my question: "Are you all right?" Moments later he stirred and appeared coherent again. I tried to get him back into bed and under the covers. After some time, he shared with me that he had fainted, and this was not the first time.

I run to clear my head. I run alone so I can pray. Usually I leave the house by 5:00 a.m., and this was a Saturday, so by the time I got to JPs I was on mile seven. Three miles to get home.

The words "you are not a doctor" began to sink in. Over the last two weeks in the evenings, I tried to really get the lay of the land: How are things going? How do you feel? What's your energy like? What did you do today? Did you go to JPs this morning? Hoping this was the one routine of his previous life that he was keeping.

JPs was part of a daily routine for Chris about nine each morning. So it was not a total surprise that this message was coming to me at a place that was central in my husband's life. I reached out and put both hands on the front window and peered inside. The shop was closed. No life there yet. But I could *see* each and every one of them all sitting together at that one table "solving the world's problems one cup at a time." These were Chris's friends and mentors—a cast of characters that were helping my husband through his darkest times. There was John and Dave, Tom and Don, Cal and Wally, Mike and possibly Jeanine. Others too joined in from time to time. They had all been there for him these past weeks. Tom had driven him to his radiation treatment, waited, and then driven him across the street to the oncology clinic where he would receive his Wednesday chemo cocktail over the course of several hours.

Then, something in my head clicked at that very moment. When was the last time he checked his blood sugar? I didn't know. Chris was responsible for all that, or was he?

Chris has type 2 diabetes and needs medication every day to keep his blood sugar levels monitored. I was thinking he just might need a slug of Gatorade like I use on my runs, but maybe these words mean I need to get one or more of his doctors involved in some decisions about his fainting spells, right away.

I probably ran the fastest 5K (3.1 miles) in my life to get home and start with that basic information. Have you taken your blood lately? I got home and found out several things that had slipped through the cracks. I was not asking some of the right questions routinely. "Yes, the nurse takes my blood each week on Wednesday when I get my chemo, and no, I haven't done it at home in a while. I gently urged him, "Why don't we do that right now." He agreed, and both of us were stunned—his blood sugar level registered 386. For those of you who don't deal with diabetes and the related consequences, 50–115 is normal, 150–180 borderline risk, and 181–380 is high, so 386 is not even on the recommended levels list.[1]

It all gets sort of fuzzy to determine which doctor trumps the others for what situations. Nobody tells you. There is no guidebook for this. So, at six thirty on a Saturday morning, I started with his oncologist, simply because I didn't know where to start, and I had just heard, *You are not a doctor.*

It took a few different times of being put on hold and then came the familiar "leave a message at the tone." Now we had to wait for the on-call physician to get back to us. How long would that be? During this wait I found out so much. "No, I'm not taking Metformin anymore because Dr. Gribben told me to stop taking it because of the chemo treatments," he said. Chris is very literal, so when a doctor says to do something, he generally adheres to that directive. How did this all start to get away from me?

The phone rang. It was the on-call oncologist practicing with Dr. Gribben. I went through all the standard questions he had for me. I wanted to jump right to the 386 number, but that's not how it all works. It's like hearing some of the 911 recordings and you want to come out of your seat. You want to cut right to the chase: "My daughter is not breathing," and he asks, "how long has she not been breathing." Send help, now! Don't ask me fourteen questions first.

We finally did get to the 386-blood level reading, and he said, "Get him to the closest emergency room, now. *He is at coma levels.*"

This was the day that I became the caregiver.

CHAPTER 14

HOSPITAL

A hospital bed is a parked taxi with the meter running.
—Groucho Marx

Healing is a matter of time, but it is sometimes
also a matter of opportunity.
—Hippocrates

Now I know why people overuse and abuse our health care system. When you are unsure of what to do, it's easy just to go to the emergency room. But this was not that case. A diabetic coma is a life-threatening complication that causes unconsciousness. When you have diabetes, dangerously high blood sugar or dangerously low blood sugar can lead to a diabetic coma.

If you lapse into a coma, you're alive, but you can't awaken or respond purposefully to sights, sounds, or other types of stimulation. Left untreated, a diabetic coma can be fatal.[1] We were in a real emergency.

Our local hospital has some of the most well-trained professionals who provide a first impression of peace, calm, and confidence, but when the situation is life-threatening, you wonder why all those questions can't be asked later. *Let's hurry this intake process along so that he can get in front of a physician immediately.* I just knew things would improve dramatically if we could get some fluids and some insulin into him.

The emergency physician was just the ticket. He asked what I thought were vital questions for the proper diagnosis, but, more importantly, we could see action. An IV had been started within minutes. With some fluids in his body and some insulin coursing through his veins, he began to perk up, and rather quickly. But not before some pretty tense moments. The doctor was trying to rule out if he had had a stroke. Chris was convinced this would be his last day on earth—he was surely going to die today. We talked briefly about the impending birth of our granddaughter to arrive in June. He was sure that he would never get to meet her face-to-face.

I was frantically trying to keep everyone notified of the changes to his health and what our next steps would be. Then I got a text from Geoff, "we are coming up right now." This was a most welcome diversion. It completely changed the mood in the room. He had something to live for, to look forward to. He began to put energy back into staying alive. The will to survive can be the game changer. *The power to harness your will makes all the difference between life and death.*

Chris can woo others. It is described as winning others over. He spent much of his career in the radio business—on-air, in sales, and in management. His career started in 1974 at a very small-town radio station in Windom, Minnesota. Let's just suffice it to say that Chris was bigger, or thought he was bigger, than Windom, Minnesota, so he took his talents a few miles down the road to Mason City, Iowa. He has a great combination of sports knowledge, along with being articulate, having a quick wit, and keeping things on time, on formula, and on queue. This is a perfect combination for an on-air radio personality and a sports play-by-play guy.

He was using all these skills, along with his woo, to convince the doctor he should go home, though just a few hours earlier his mood was somber. The past week had been very difficult. February's temperatures and snowfall were adding weight onto an already difficult journey. We had to call in the cavalry on Wednesday morning just to get him to the radiation facility, and then chemo treatment after that. This would be the last chemotherapy treatment, and Chris was committed to being on time and on formula. Our small neighborhood streets had not been plowed by the time he needed to leave. There were high levels of anxiety, to be sure. We didn't even want to try getting through ten inches of unplowed snow, so we asked a friend with an SUV to drive him two blocks to where another friend who already had volunteered to take him that day was waiting. During those last few weeks, Chris was "the package." His friends were committed to getting the package to its destination, through wind, snow, sleet, and bitter cold.

The ER doctor was leaning toward admitting him, and Chris would have none of it. "I'm going home. I'm good." He had to show the doctor that he had recovered his strength and his balance. Around the halls and corridors of the emergency room he went, with a pace I hadn't even seen in the healthiest of times. "One more lap," the doctor asked. And Chris delivered. We were being released to go back home.

You know how it goes when you've been through a harrowing situation. You want others to hear the blow-by-blow commentary. We replayed all that when Geoff and Ellen arrived. On that day they practiced *presence*. Nothing more. The visit to the emergency room, the potential talk of a stroke, all the prescribed procedures to get a handle on the complete situation, and injections galore left Chris exhausted. His normal sleep pattern was about twenty hours a day. He needed his rest, and I needed real people, talking real life issues. They were having a baby. How wonderful is that.

Geoff and Ellen's visit was so therapeutic for me. The flavor from the fish and chips I ordered at Chequers in Saugatuck still lingers deep in my memory. We sat at the corner table right next to the fireplace. I welcomed the warmth of the fire with the smell of the wood and the movement and mystique of the flames. We talked about their dreams, hopes, and future with this new little person they would call their daughter.

What can you do to help caregivers? Get them out of the house. Take them to a restaurant. Ask about their needs. Let them talk. Really listen to them so they will feel real. Make the topic of your conversations relatively benign or vanilla. Don't make it heavy. Lighten their load. Practice presence. Be with them, and then leave.

*I praise you because I am
fearfully and wonderfully made;
your works are wonderful,
I know that full well.*

Psalm 139:14

PART 4
KNOW THE PATIENT

CHAPTER 15
THRIVING TO HEAL

*The cactus thrives in the desert, while
the fern thrives in the wetland.*
—Vera Nazarian

The most common form of despair is not being who you are.
—Søren Kierkegaard

After the initial diagnosis I searched the internet sporadically for details and for answers. I am sure I was looking for others who had been through the journey we were now on. "Cancer. It is an uncontrolled growth of abnormal cells. Cancer develops when the body's normal control mechanism stops working. Old cells do not die, and cells grow out of control, forming new, abnormal cells. These extra cells form a mass of tissue called a tumor."[1]

One woman started a blog and shared many details, but then her husband died. I really didn't want to read that one anymore. The University of Michigan site had details that were uncomfortable to read. The stories were quite graphic, very real, but mostly unsettling. I would not be able to share these with Chris. However, they were all success stories.

I had been reading about Brian Tracy, who also was diagnosed with throat cancer, but in 2010. Mr. Tracy is a well-known author, speaker, and motivator. Over the years, I have read some of his books. Mr. Tracy started his treatment plan in April 2010 and continued his speaking schedule through April and May. He then started six weeks of radiation treatment in August and was back addressing small and large audiences all over the world in September. It appeared from what I was reading that the process for him was quite easy. This was positive and very promising, but Chris now found solace only in his chair. I couldn't even imagine him getting dressed and driving in to work.

Jim Kelly, retired quarterback for the Buffalo Bills, and Chris Mortensen, analyst for ESPN, were also actively battling throat cancer at the same time as Chris. I searched for anything I could find on their current status and recovery. I had a desire to know more, especially anything positive that could give us hope. I kept a lot of what I learned to myself. This passage came to mind when I'd find something important but something that potentially would only create more anxiety: "but Mary treasured up all these things and pondered them in her heart" (Luke 2:19). I realized this journey ultimately was going to be ours alone. There was no consistent recipe like the one I have for our highly requested lasagna. We would not be handed a script. There were going to be no exacts. I was discovering very quickly that this experience would be highly personalized, probably not replicated, and ultimately the greatest human endeavor we had undertaken so far in our lives together. We would need to be a great team. We would need to practice what we teach.

What we have been teaching is to know yourself and the power that greater levels of self-awareness can bring. Self-awareness is the ability to monitor your thoughts, emotions, and actions from moment to moment. It is knowing, understanding, and feeling comfortable in your own DNA. It includes being clear about what you like and what you don't like. We simply need to know ourselves more because it is a mechanism for self-control, and this allows you to gain greater mastery over your choices. While self-awareness in the workplace is profound and essential, there is nothing more profound than self-awareness for life—your very life. But self-reflection is hard work, and we all have blind spots. Lack of self-awareness is a common root cause of disease, stress, and unrest. In her book *The Happiness Project*, Gretchen Rubin says, "You can choose what you do, but you can't choose what you like to do." She goes on to say, "The tougher code to crack is how to become more self-aware."[2]

Great tools facilitate self-reflection. We don't want to do a flyby in understanding ourselves; we want to do a deep dive. As a Kolbe Certified™ Master Team Consultant and practitioner, I believe that the Kolbe A™ Index is among the greatest tools to help us do just that. It allows us to look at the "trinity of self-awareness"—know yourself, improve yourself, and complement yourself.

I am drawn to it because it provides consistent language to understand our innate striving patterns. It helps understand that outward behaviors and actions are triggered by our innate needs. These innate needs are ingrained in people; therefore, they are predictable and reliable. We can trust them. We can count on people to operate to their true self.[3] We know in advance what people will need to do—what they will strive at or seek out to do.

This innate force is at the foundation of how we strive as human beings. Striving is tied to our productivity. Our health, happiness, satisfaction, and fulfillment all are tied to our striving. So too is stress. The essential piece is how effectively we can manage our striving instincts or striving energy.

William James, often referred to as the father of American psychology, said in 1887: "Instinct is usually defined as the faculty of acting in such a way as to produce certain ends, without foresight of the ends, and without previous education in the performance."[4]

These striving instincts trigger how we use our time. Energy and time are connected. If I have certain striving energy, I will use my time more naturally doing specific actions or tasks. If I don't have certain striving instincts, I will put off, resist, or avoid doing specific actions. There is a common saying we might hear often: "I don't have time for that." What likely is truer is that "I don't have the energy to do that." It's not really time; it's energy. So, energy, not time, is our most precious resource. When we are using our energy well, there is a sense of effortlessness.

This knowledge is a foundational tool in the workplace because it provides teams with a common operating frame of reference and communication language. It promotes greater self-awareness, better understanding of others, and an ability to recognize the cause of conflict between people. It provides understanding, knowledge, and guidance to minimize the negative effects of this conflict, how to improve relationships and get along with others, and ultimately how to improve communication and interactions to elevate team performance.

Through the awareness that comes from the suite of Kolbe Indexes, we can live more productive, satisfying, peaceful, and calmer lives. It is a piece of wisdom that might save our busy generation. This understanding will enable you to be more inner-directed, self-referring, and true to yourself. It is a tool that unlocks the mystery of life and relationships. It is a piece of wisdom we feel everyone should have. As a marital team we have utilized this insight consistently, but once the diagnosis was confirmed, we had a heightened sense that this would be the intangible advantage that would help us with the critical teamwork that would be so necessary. We put the twenty-four years of self-awareness about our striving needs into intentional practice every day. So, if we had this wisdom for twenty-four years, then why did Chris get sick? I can't answer that question. I do not know. One day a cell goes rogue. But since we have this wisdom, we want to help others.

Busyness is our status symbol today. But a busy life is not necessarily a life well lived. Our busyness and expectations of ourselves do not always align with our natural tendencies, and this causes stress. Experts on stress define it as "a condition or feeling experienced when a person perceives that demands exceed the personal and social resources the individual is able to mobilize."[5] Hans Selye, an esteemed endocrinologist, defined it as "a non-specific response of the body to a demand." Today, the American Institute of Stress says that stress is the number one health issue in America.[6] Stress causes disease. It's that simple.

To understand the innate necessities for individuals who are in the healing process is huge. I realized very early on that if Chris was going to heal, we needed to minimize what he naturally resisted. "A person who is at peace, surrounded by loving support, will quite literally heal better, drawing on the resources of body, mind and spirit."[7] For Chris to thrive again, he needed to heal, and for him to heal, he needed to be in the environment that allowed him to thrive. If those environments are not there, it will hinder the healing process because the mind and body are using valuable energy going against the grain. I wanted Chris to be going with the grain, no matter what each day brought. I wanted him to abound again. Second Corinthians 9:8 says, "And God is able to bless you abundantly, so that in all things at all times, having all that you need, you will abound in every good work." My job would be to live out Ephesians 4:29: "Do not let any unwholesome talk come out of your mouths, but only what is helpful for building others up according to their needs, that it may benefit those who listen."

CHAPTER 16
KOLBE IS A BREAKTHROUGH

When you know someone's Kolbe, you can refresh them.
—Dan Broekhuizen

Understand the laws of your own nature.
—Gretchen Rubin

Rarely do we see a real breakthrough. However, on May 6, 1954, an English runner, Roger Bannister, made a significant breakthrough—the first man to break the four-minute-mile barrier.

Breaking that barrier had been a goal for runners for centuries. Back in Greece, coaches tried some pretty strange tactics to speed up their runners. One was to release wild animals to chase the runners, forcing them to run faster or be attacked. Another was to feed them tiger's milk. None of these tactics worked, so experts decided that man's body was simply not designed to run that fast. But on that historic day in May, Roger Bannister proved the doctors, trainers, and experts wrong. And then, thirty-seven runners broke the four-minute mile in the following year. And in 1956, three hundred runners accomplished the same feat. It took just one man to do it, and the rest believed.[1]

On October 12, 2019, Eliud Kipchoge, a thirty-four-year-old runner from Kenya, broke the two-hour barrier for a marathon. The run organized specifically for him to break this barrier featured an electric pacer car that shot a laser beam to mark the best position on the road. In addition, forty-one professional runners rotated running alongside him to set his pace.[2] It is not recognized as an official record, but sixty-five years after Roger Bannister made his mark on the world, Kipchoge was jubilant about the effort and all those who helped him accomplish it with these words: "I want to inspire many people, that no human is limited."

I see the development of the Kolbe suite of assessment tools for self-awareness on par with this breakthrough. In 1988, Kathy Kolbe developed a proven and reliable tool to assess what people will do, what they won't do, and what they are willing to do. What we "can" do is altogether different. We can do anything we set our minds to do, but we need to recognize the level of pain this may cause. This self-awareness tool is designed to help all of us understand our sweet spot when it comes to taking action. It describes how we will strive toward a goal. It provides personal language on how we each "get things done." It is separate and distinct from our intelligence or our personality type.

This is a breakthrough for everyone, and everyone needs to know their Kolbe MO (mode of operation). Because this is the foundation of our work, it was natural to apply these principles directly to our health crisis to *cut out the waste* and help Chris *carry only what was essential* for him.

Kolbe provides understanding and gives language for the environment each person will need to thrive, the type of communication that will resonate with his or her needs, and the best way for the person to handle specific tasks and requirements that this diagnosis may bring. This insight creates a powerful advantage in the face of adversity.

Kolbe measures four striving instincts that we all share universally: the instinct to probe, the instinct to pattern, the instinct to improvise, and the instinct to demonstrate.

12 Kolbe Strengths™

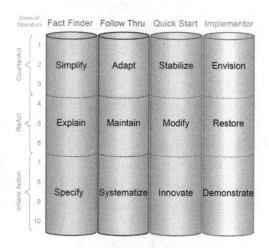

Each person has levels or zones to which he or she will use each of those four instincts. At the 1–3 level, we will literally counteract the instinct. For example, someone who is a 1–3 in the probing instinct will look for the bottom line first before inquiring, investigating, and probing. It also means that a person will naturally resist or avoid operating this way.

At the 4–6 level, or zone of operation, a person will respond by assisting and helping to further actions that result from that instinct. Someone like me who is a 4 in the instinct to probe will go along with others' research, will look for data and details that are already out there, and will recognize, piggyback, support, and rely on someone else's information, facts, and due diligence. Researching in-depth creates stress for me.

At the 7–10 zone, a person will initiate or insist on actions that result from that instinct. This is where he or she needs to begin solving the problem. It is how the person will use his or her time and energy first to tackle the issue or the challenge. As a 9 in the instinct to improvise, I don't fold in a crisis; I embrace it.

Action Modes®
As Defined by Kathy Kolbe

Fact Finder	Fact Finder is the instinctive need to probe and the way we gather and share information. When people operate at a 7-10 level it leads to actions where individuals will research, analyze, study, justify, debate, assess, prove, detail, and document. Chris is a 7; I am a 4.
Follow Thru	Follow Thru is the instinctive need to pattern and the way we organize and design. When people operate at the 7-10 level it leads to actions where an individual will create a sense of order, structure, organize, systematize, plan, coordinate, arrange, schedule, and complete. Chris is a 7; I am a 2.
Quick Start	Quick Start is the instinctive need to improvise and the way we deal with risk and uncertainty. When people operate at the 7-10 zone it leads to actions where an individual will experiment, deviate, change, invent, risk, shortcut, originate, brainstorm, and challenge. Chris is a 5; I am a 9.
Implementor	Implementor is the instinctive need to demonstrate and the way we handle space and tangibles. When people operate at the 7-10 zone it leads to actions where an individual will construct, build, practice, put together, move, use physical effort, show, transport, and deal with mechanics. Chris is a 2; I am a 4.

To learn more about Action Modes® or other Kolbe Corp Material, visit
ComeHomeAliveBook.com

Mari Martin
Kolbe A™ Result

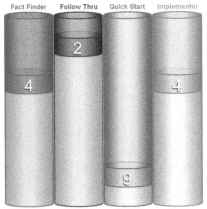

Chris Martin
Kolbe A™ Result

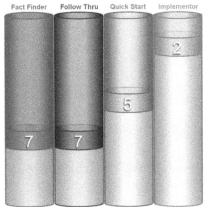

As individuals, we are propelled by these creative forces. Understanding these innate forces, even though they may be dormant and are merely potential during a time of sickness and ill health, is essential in getting people to begin striving again and on their way to thriving.

The Kolbe A Index takes only minutes to complete online, and the current cost is fifty-five dollars. Both the patient and the caregiver should complete these separately. One should not answer for the other. To learn more about the Kolbe A Index and other Kolbe Corp. material, visit comehomealivebook.com. Kolbe Corp. says this about the Kolbe A: "It helps you understand your conative attributes and sets you on a path to joyfully tackle the challenges you might face in your personal and professional life."[3]

When people get the results back, they are amazed at the accuracy. This is what we hear:

- "You have nailed it! I can't believe how accurate this is. This is how I operate," or
- "I always knew this about myself but found it difficult to explain to others. You have given me the vocabulary to share with others what works best for me. What a gift."

There is a joke about a preacher who dies in the downpour that turns into a flood. It goes something like this:

A storm descends upon a small town, and the downpour turns into a flood. As the waters rise, the local preacher kneels in prayer on the church porch, surrounded by water. By and by, one of the locals comes up the street in a canoe.

"Better get in, Preacher. The waters are rising fast."

"No," says the preacher. "I have faith in the Lord. He will save me."

Still the waters rise. Now the preacher is up on the balcony, wringing his hands in supplication, when another guy zips up in a motorboat.

"Come on, Preacher. We need to get you out of here. The levee's gonna break any minute."

Once again, the preacher is unmoved. "I shall remain. The Lord will see me through."

After a while the levee breaks, and the flood rushes over the church until only the steeple remains above water. The preacher is up there, clinging to the cross, when a helicopter descends out of the clouds, and a state trooper calls down to him through a megaphone.

"Grab the ladder, Preacher. This is your last chance."

Once again, the preacher insists the Lord will deliver him.

And predictably, he drowns.[4]

So often we are looking for celestial answers and miss out on the everyday lifelines of a canoe, a boat, and a helicopter. Kolbe is not a miracle. It is not faith or prayer, or belief or gratitude expressed to God. But it is something I firmly believe God has worked through Kathy Kolbe to develop, to help each of us through our unique life journey. Be on the lookout for the right circumstances, the right message, and the right people to come into your life—a flat tire, a newspaper article, a conversation with a friend over coffee.

As a caregiver, know your loved one's love language. This can be done through the love languages detailed in Gary Chapman's book *The 5 Love Languages*.[5] The five love languages are: Words of Affirmation, Quality Time, Receiving Gifts, Acts of Service, and Physical Touch. Mine is Physical Touch. When I am hurting, I want someone to reach out and touch me. This instantly lets me know that I am loved. Chris's is Quality Time and Words of Affirmation. "Tell me I'm doing well with my medication and following the doctor's orders. Be with me. Hang out with me even though my breath is bad, and I can't get out of my chair." I would work my way into his chair with him and share what happened throughout the day. We would talk about little things. I would try not to correct or admonish in any way but reinforce positive words like the ones from Dr. Edlund: "your tumor is melting like ice off a hot tin roof." He'd hold onto me and provide the physical touch I needed. I felt like I could get up and do it all again tomorrow. The power truly is in the knowing.

CHAPTER 17
ACTING ON WHAT YOU KNOW

*It's not what you know, but what you do
with what you know, you know?*
—*Anonymous*

It's what you learn after you know it all that counts.
—*John Wooden*

Chris's Kolbe MO is 7 7 5 2. This means that Chris needs to have a strategy and a plan to manage his day-to-day activities smoothly. He needs specific information, and he needs proof and evidence that his doctors were prescribing a plan that had worked in the past. Chris thrives when he can get into a routine. Chris needs to bring structure and predictability to his surroundings when faced with crisis or chaotic situations. When Chris has a plan, a map, and a course laid out that he can replicate, this creates positive energy for him. He needs the spaces around him to be neat, tidy, and orderly. He craves consistency and consolidation. When faced with uncertainty, Chris is willing to try new approaches, but only if there is a rhyme and a reason for doing so. He's willing to modify plans if he must, and he is open to finding alternatives and making adjustments as new information surfaces. But Chris is all thumbs when he must work with his hands to open bandages or crush his medication, as he could no longer take his pills orally.

One of the hardest decisions Chris made was to have a feeding tube inserted into his stomach wall. This type of cancer required the feeding tube because the radiation would kill off the good cells along with the tumorous cells in his throat. Many of us just take for granted the process of eating. For those undergoing radiation treatments in the throat area, the entire mouth is in pain, and the saliva glands are destroyed, rendering most foods difficult to chew and virtually impossible to swallow. Thank goodness his sister was first to respond when we discussed the feeding tube by saying, "That will just be the greatest thing." It gave him a sense that others had survived before with this, and it was no big deal.

Every meal he would sit at the kitchen table, and arrayed in front of him was his "science lab." A huge challenge was that this task required him to handle things, tear things, manipulate things, and work with his hands. This forced him to go against his grain. He would have to muster energy he did not have naturally. It exhausted him just to look at all the physical things that were on the kitchen table—beaker, stir sticks, spoons, glass, water, nutrition, syringe, needles, tube. *And now I have to make all this work with my hands?* No matter how hard you try, you cannot consistently operate in a way that is inconsistent with who you are. Going against your grain will not be sustainable. *Teamwork is critical.*

Dr. Timothy Paterick, my high school classmate and cardiologist now practicing at Aurora BayCare Medical Center in Green Bay, Wisconsin, says in his recent book *Invest in Yourself,* "Our doctor cannot help us unless we help ourselves. When you have the freedom to do things in your own way, this allows you to adapt to the infinite complexities of life."[1]

So why do we get cancer, you ask? Did I do something wrong? "'Neither this man nor his parents sinned,' said Jesus, 'but this happened so that the works of God might be displayed in him.'" (John 9:3) Life is a test. Maybe the test really was mine.

CHAPTER 18

UNKNOWNS, AMBIGUITIES, COMPLICATIONS

A hero is somebody who voluntarily walks into the unknown.
—Tom Hanks

Sometimes you find yourself in the middle of nowhere, and sometimes in the middle of nowhere you find yourself.
—Edward Fallon

W hat good is all this research around the cure, if as humans our bodies are unable to adapt, and we can't handle and manage the cure? What good is the cure if, in the end, the cure is the killer?

2/23/2014

From: Mari Martin

To: All medical personnel involved with Chris Martin and his current treatments

Chris went to the emergency room on 2/22/2014 because of dizziness and a fainting spell he had about

2:00 a.m. He has been very lethargic since Wednesday of last week when he did not take much nutrition through the feeding tube on that day. Things seemed to go downhill from there.

He was released from the ER on 2/22/2014 to the care of his PCP, Patrick Hulst. This is just to update all of you on the situation that is occurring since then.

He did not tolerate much via the feeding tube for the remainder of 2/22. I encouraged him to take water via the tube, but he was very reluctant. We were able to get four cans of nutrition in him, but the evening feeding was exceedingly difficult, and he vomited most of that up.

At 5:00 a.m. on 2/23/2014 his FBS was 257. He is not very coherent. He is very reluctant to take even water via the feeding tube. I have given him at most 6 oz. of water via the tube and 2 oz. of formula. When I try giving formula, he immediately is nauseated and needs to vomit. He is resting comfortably, and I am trying to give him 2 oz. of water about every 30 minutes. That is the current situation.

I have just spoken with the on-call Dr. from Thomas Gribben's office and he advised I take Chris back to the Emergency Room. We are headed there now.

This hospital stay proved to be very valuable. Chris learned a new way to feed through the tube. The nurse called it "gravity feeding." It would take more time, but the stomach naturally let the fluids in instead of being forced. He felt encouraged that he could do it himself. To heal, he needed more fluids and more calories. It was great in theory; now we had to get home in our natural environment and put it into practice. Dr. Gribben called the seven chemo treatments that he had already received "good," with no more rounds of chemo to go. A milestone. The chemo portion was over and done. He had successfully finished that part of the journey. I could see a lift in his spirit and a renewed commitment to make the new feeding approach work.

It was late February. While Chris had a revived outlook and greater motivation, I was dealing with exceptionally brutal winter conditions. Along with caring for Chris and my full-time work, I was now the main attraction for snow removal. There were days when all went well, and I could get the snowblower started. And then there were days when I'd cry out in frustration because I just didn't have the strength to pull the cord hard and fast at the same time. The snow was getting so high the arc of the thrower was too low, and the snow would come tumbling right back down on the area that I had just cleared. I vividly remember screaming at the top of my lungs in the garage in total frustration. The wind was howling. It was freezing, and the snow would just not let up. I went into the house and took off my boots, hat, scarf, balaclava (it was brutally cold), gloves, coat, and ski pants. I quieted my heart and prayed for the snow blower to start. It was a very selfish prayer. But it is what I needed at that moment. *Don't pretty it up.* I was determined this snow, this wind, and the below-zero temperatures were not going to get in the way. I put everything back on and stomped back out to the garage. With one pull, the engine revved, and the snowblower responded. This was a very visible answer to prayer. The God that I trusted was in command.

On Tuesday of that week, Chris was released from the hospital, and on Thursday, he resumed his radiation treatments. Dr. Edlund was very encouraged in spite of the recent setbacks. Only three more radiation treatments left—Friday, Monday, and Tuesday. He was on the home stretch. Chris was sure that he could make it now. His treatment protocol would be done. He would finish well; of this I was certain.

Friday was a great diversion. We were having our photos taken professionally for our new website. Both the photographer and the advertising agency people were all hanging out at our location—an older home in the heart of Hope College's campus area. We had done business with TheImageGroup over the years, so it was great to see some familiar faces, joke around, and get our minds off cancer. It was fun to plan for the wardrobe changes. We had to figure out how we coordinated with each other. Chris had brought a snappy black jacket that made his gray hair pop. He was much thinner, but overall, on the outside he did look healthy. No one, I'm sure, thought he was close to death. I could see all the effort was a struggle, but he put on his game face and made it through. I am so glad we have those photos from that day.

I believed that once Chris was through this stretch, we would begin to see weight gain, recovery, and an overall visage of "Hey, you're looking good." This was not the case for Chris. The scariest times for us came after the treatment plan was over.

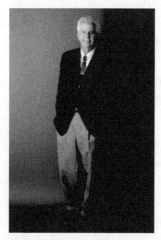 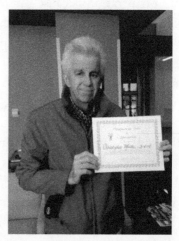

Photo taken by Rob Walcott   *Last day of treatment—*
four days later

CHAPTER 19
THE LIFELINE OF HUMILITY

If you are never scared, embarrassed or hurt,
it means you never take chances.
—Julia Soul

But I learned that there's a certain character that can be built
from embarrassing yourself endlessly. If you can sit happy with
embarrassment, there's not much else that can really get to ya.
—Christian Bale

Our bodily functions are the human stories that get told over and over again, especially by children. It makes them giggle nervously and brings embarrassment the color of a stop sign. There are many stories along the way of awkward, scary, and sensitive moments for Chris. Most of those have to do with his feeding tube.

We met an amazing guide named Antoinella on our family trip to Italy in 2001. Antoinella's most famous words as we all poured onto the motor coach at six thirty in the morning were, "Wakey, wakey." Some people, as you can imagine, rebelled when they heard those words day after day. On the day we were to drive the most miles, from Florence down to Naples, she made the miles go by quicker with her countless stories about Italian mothers and their sons and the quirky, unique relationships that evolve in their culture. After she had the entire bus roaring with laughter that leaves your stomach sore, one passenger asked, "Now, tell us about the bidet." Without missing a beat, Antoinella said, "That is a story for another day."

And so goes the story of the feeding tube. I have several graphic memories of this means that literally saved Chris's life. But for Chris, this perhaps brings up the most emotion. He knows that without it, he simply would not have survived. His sister gave him the necessary boost by saying, "This will just be the greatest thing." With those words tucked close, he went for the procedure to have it inserted into his stomach. It is done at an outpatient surgery facility with a little bit of "numbing up." There is a tinge of pressure when the tube is inserted and then a balloon secures the tube to the inside of the stomach wall. There are no bandages, and there is no bleeding.

Chris was not sure exactly what to expect. He simply had no expectations and had not done any preliminary research. Along with his sister, Dr. Edlund insisted, "Get the feeding tube." He didn't realize how emotional a decision this would be, especially to a very vain man. He left the facility that day with a fifteen-inch tube hanging out of his stomach. All he could think of was, "This is just prolonging it. I'm a goner." He had already lost about forty pounds, was not feeling well, did not have an appetite, and now was going to need to feed himself this way. Despair set in. I'm sure he felt like crawling into a corner in hopes that he could just die like a dog.

Getting used to the tube was a big learning curve. This was how he would need to get the fluids and the nutrition that would give him the proper energy to stay in the fight. He was very protective and self-conscious of it. He didn't want to bang it or hit it wrong, otherwise he thought it might bleed. He imagined it somehow becoming dislodged, and then kept to himself what he imagined would happen if it did. There were days when dark thoughts crept in, and he stared down at his stomach and said, "I am on life support, the end is near." This tube was there to provide a bridge, or alternate process, while he couldn't eat normally. The key word to remember is "while." But it also was requiring him to use Implementor energy that was not innate. Seven times a day he was needing to do that which he naturally resisted. He had to focus the job by going at it through his natural strength—Follow

Thru. He needed to make it a routine—a specific time, a regular pattern, a process, a formula. He remembers, "I was getting accustomed to it but fighting it every step of the way."

Eating this way has no sensation. There is no taste, so therefore, no enjoyment. Plus, seven times each day he would have to set up the "science lab." When there's no taste and no enjoyment, how do you get motivated to crush your medication, fill the beaker with thirty-two ounces of water, flush the tube with the water, begin the feeding by taking in water, mix the crushed medications with the water, take in the nutrition, take in more water, and flush the tube to finish? He absolutely hated the process.

When he switched to the gravity approach, he would have to wait, and wait and wait until his stomach accepted the fluids in the tube. He tired very easily from the process. I wasn't there during the day, so I couldn't observe his true intake of water and nutrition. When I was home, and on the weekends, I was ready to serve him by taking on all the Implementor work—crushing the pills, filling, holding, making, handling, hauling, moving. Whatever physical activity was necessary to smooth out the kinks, that's how I saw that I could help and support him. I also could watch and observe the process, and try to minimize anything that Chris might see as embarrassing. This was our new normal whether we liked it or not.

I have two distinct memories of the feeding tube. The first was in the parking lot of the University of Michigan Hospital during a visit to see Dr. Prince. If Chris was forced to go outside of his routine and pattern, his instinct was to avoid. Just not do it. So, he'd avoid that feeding. By this time, we understood all too well the impact of his fluid intake. Avoiding "the meal" would be harmful to him. But how were we supposed to lay out all the equipment necessary in the front seats and dashboard of the car. His car was always immaculate. Not a spot of dirt, not an extra piece of paper, nothing extraneous was ever in his car. Now, we were going to clutter it up with syringes, a beaker, pills, cups, cans of nutrition. Not on your life. There were times when we traveled the night before and stayed in a hotel, for just this reason—to have a place to properly set up the science lab in private. On this day we had no private hotel room. It was going to be the car or nothing.

It was quite the battle. But in the end, we did it together. We parked in a very remote area that was the farthest from the entry doors and finished the job. The atmosphere between the two of us was not warm and fuzzy, but Chris can commit to getting it finished and bringing things to closure. That was the focus we had to take when circumstances were unusual or awkward.

The other distinct memory was in the parking lot of the famous golf course in Pinehurst, North Carolina—Pinehurst No. 2. It was our vacation in September 2014. Only this time we were not in a healthcare facility but one of the most revered places on earth. We were in a dignified space. Golfers from all over the world come to Pinehurst No. 2. Who might drive in and park next to us? And to add to that atmosphere, it was a very hot day. Hot, humid, and muggy.

Again, after a heated conversational battle—okay, let's call it a fight, because it was one—we managed the twenty odd minutes of pain to work through the process. What is always an unknown is whether things will flow smoothly through the tube or there will be backups, clogs, and overflows. An overflow in the car would be a catastrophe. This is why it is much easier just to bypass the feeding. From Chris's perspective: "I don't need it anyway, and let's just get on with seeing this golf course we drove all this way to see."

During these twenty minutes, several employees started coming in for their shifts. Little did we know that where we were parked out in the back forty is exactly the area that the staff used for parking. I am sure that more than one of those young people walked past our car with their eyebrows raised. What are those people over there doing? Yes, it was very hot and muggy outside. We didn't have the car running with nice cool air pulsing out the vents. The windows were steaming up. We were sure at any moment management was going to come out and demand that we vacate this distinguished property. Certainly, we were riffraff.

But it was also on this very vacation that Chris showed off his tube while walking on the beach one afternoon. He had come full circle for the most part and accepted that this was his life now. He knows that "I am alive because of it. It is what it is. If you want to laugh and poke fun of me, well then go ahead. I'll laugh along with you."

We headed out for a walk on the beach with his fifteen-inch feeding tube stuck down the front of his bathing suit. When a small child pointed and said, "Mommy, mommy, that man has a funny tube coming out of his stomach," we smiled, looked at each other, joined hands, and enjoyed every step, every breath, every piece of warmth and sunshine down the white, sandy beach of Myrtle Beach, South Carolina.

Chris would ultimately have three different tubes. Just like tires that get old and lose their traction, so it goes with a feeding tube. It needs to be replaced. He went into the hospital again as an outpatient. The nurse asked if he'd like something to numb the pain and he said no. This is how the replacement process went. The existing tube was just pulled out. Pop, out it went! The doctor took the new one and stuffed it in. That was it—a no-brainer procedure. The second one was just like the first, about fifteen inches. But the third one was flush to his body.

By this time, he and the tube were on speaking terms. You might even say they were becoming friends. He was back to syringing the nutrition in and forcing the fluids into his stomach. His body was accepting and complying. There were no more battles. It was his routine. It was his lifeline.

For we are God's handiwork, created in Christ Jesus to do good works, which God prepared in advance for us to do.

Ephesians 2:10

PART 5
KNOW THE CAREGIVER

CHAPTER 20
KNOW YOUR MODUS OPERANDI (MO)

My friend ... care for your psyche ... know thyself, for once we know ourselves, we may learn how to care for ourselves.
—*Socrates*

It's not the load that breaks you down.
It's the way you carry it.
—*Lena Horne*

My Kolbe MO is 4 2 9 4. The first 4 means that I React or respond in the instinct to probe, called the Fact Finder Action Mode. This means I will help research, but initiating research will take me out of my comfort zone. Right after Chris's diagnosis, my first response was that I would not be researching for hours on the internet about his situation. Oh, I did some at first, but it truly exhausts me. It's much more natural to work with what someone else has researched. Writing this book is a stretch for me, but I so believe that others need to know the facts and realize that we must do more prevention to stop this disease and the current inhumane treatment protocol. My best efforts come when I can explain things to others, and hopefully with just the right amount of detail—not too much/not too little.

The 2 means that I CounterAct in the instinct to pattern, called the Follow Thru Action Mode. It means I look for ways to improve on a system. It means forcing me to operate according to rigid systems or rituals will be met with resistance. It's best if others just tell me what needs to be done and then leave me alone to figure out the how. Give me a set of directions, and I will most certainly be looking for the alternate route. You can guess that if I use the navigation system in my car, I will not follow it exactly to the finish line. There always seems to be a better, quicker, shorter way. Any kind of task that I must repeat again and again will get boring. I have left or changed jobs precisely because of this; I just didn't know it at the time. I must be especially intentional when taking medication according to the directions. I've had to set the doses out on the counter to ensure I take what the doctor prescribes each day. It also means that I will switch tasks frequently without the need to bring closure to each one in sequence. Sequential is how Chris needs to operate, and I need just the opposite. I need sporadic and random. I don't have a need to keep things in order, make things neat and tidy, and put things back where they belong. I have a need to keep things out and accessible. This is a more productive work environment for me. But this natural randomness that I need creates intense stress for him. This has been our greatest marital dilemma, and it would come to its full exposure as I became his primary caregiver.

In the Follow Thru striving mode, Chris is a 7 and I am a 2. I counteract what he initiates. Swell. It would be so helpful if all of us knew these natural striving mechanisms that we have before we get married. I often think, wouldn't it be wonderful if we all had a bar code on our foreheads before we fall hopelessly in love. I see this difference as "jumping two fences." It's easier to relate to people when your zones of operation are right next door. Ours were attuned to jumping over the Grand Canyon. In organizing systems where Chris naturally initiates, I resist. I might even say that I prevent it. Think about the precise environment you are trying to create that allows you to thrive, only to have someone in the same household come along and stomp it to pieces. This is how things were before Kolbe. After Kolbe we had so much greater awareness, but we weren't in a life-or-death situation, until now.

I realized if he was to *trim out the waste and carry just what was necessary*, I would need to be intentional about keeping our home free of clutter. Please don't think we live in a junk heap. It most certainly is not. There are just times when everything is not perfectly organized and in its place as Chris would like. What does my closet look like today, thirty years later? It's better. But it will never be perfectly organized. I just can't sustain that because I would constantly need to be rearranging the order of the closet. In my mind, that is a huge waste of time. I was literally sick to my stomach when reading the mega bestseller, *The Life-Changing Magic of Tidying Up.*[1]

I began a practice of creating "lanes" where I could collect things in one place that needed to be put away. If something needed to go to the bedroom upstairs, then I would put it on the corner of the counter near the staircase heading upstairs. If I was going upstairs, then I'd look on the counter, and magically those were whisked away and taken to where they belonged. Physical things (using my 4 in Implementor) are easier to put away than paper. Filing and sorting are an intense effort. Being able to decide what mail should be thrown away immediately has always plagued me. Paper and mail tend to build up and spread on a surface. Our son, Geoff, who is also a 2 in Follow Thru calls it, "his horizontal filing system." I discovered that I could put things "on" easier than put things "away." I acquired a jewelry tree. What a marvelous invention for people like me. Now each piece of jewelry had a place. Again, I would use my "lanes" either upstairs or downstairs to get things first on the proper floor of our home and then to get them in their place. As a 2 in Follow Thru, I can get things in their place, just not right away, or according to someone else's timing. Think of it as a piecemeal effort. It might be the last thing I will do, while this is the first thing Chris will do. Chris did not have the physical energy to do it, but his brain needed this so his system could naturally concentrate on healing. I could make this sustainable if I could learn to make a habit out of it. "Committing the more mundane parts of our life to habit and routine frees up RAM for the things that matter to us," says Bruce Grierson.[2] Now, in our new home, I have a room that is all mine; everything is out and accessible, and that is sacred.

The 9 means that I Initiate in the instinct to improvise, called the Quick Start Action Mode. I need environments where I can brainstorm and verbalize. This is my job. I lead team training sessions to help every member understand how every other member operates. This leads to being able to accelerate the communication, collaboration, and team-building process. It especially helps understand the root cause of conflict. I serve as a catalyst to move groups through unknown territory. So, each day, I could do that which I do best. This kept my thriving mechanism aligned completely. Talking for a living fits me perfectly. I work best with open-endedness, ambiguity, and unknowns. Deadlines are essential for me to keep on time and on task. When there is no deadline, it is hard to engage. Challenging situations are something that I run to, not away from. Something challenging needs to be on my plate, like running marathons. I am energized in situations where I need to ad lib, think on my feet, and experiment. Chris said once to me, "What I love about you is that you are never afraid, and you are always ready to go."

The last 4 means that I React in the instinct to demonstrate, called the Implementor Action Mode. This describes why I have been in this business thirty years. We want to build lasting solutions within companies. I want to help others get things working again. I will engage and respond when asked to fix things. My passion statement is: "opening lines of communication in a broken and hurting world." When I can be in the middle of those situations, I am a "hog in slop." I will definitely test ingredients when cooking. Chris's "science lab" became my challenge. I do not put off or avoid manual effort; I was willing and ready to help with all that was required. I will never forget the day he said, "It is time to stop all this." My role was to remove or minimize the physical aspects, hands-on efforts, and mechanical contraptions of this challenge. My proofs of love were to tear open the bandage and gauze wrappers, to apply when his hands no longer worked to do that, to be the pill crusher, and to readily volunteer to do the tube feedings when Chris had lost all will to keep going. Chris wants to make things look pretty; I want them to work and function. The function of something is far more important to me than how it looks. When we buy things for our home, I go more for quality and the feel; Chris will melt at the style. I want solid wood doors that have heft. I realized very early on that if Chris was going to heal, we needed to minimize having him do what he naturally resisted. I became his Implementor hands and feet. *Teammates are what you will need.*

A few years back, Dave Van Andel, who leads the Van Andel Institute in Grand Rapids, Michigan, was speaking at a Family Business

Alliance conference. He said, "if only we could find the formula for how to get along." In Kolbe we have indeed the formula to know and understand our points of difference and potential areas that will develop into conflict. I believe God is commanding us to learn tools that open the door to learning just these types of things about each other, so in our marriages and in our relationships, we can keep the focus on the saving grace represented in Christ dying for our sins. Staying focused on this gift of salvation allows us to die to ourselves, while still staying nourished and not giving up our own selfhood.

"Marriage is so personal that no one is able to stand outside of another relationship to see why they bond. And don't expect everyone to see what you see in each other that cleaves and sticks you together."[3] Couples oftentimes divorce when they have no tools to navigate their differences. The buildup of these differences leads to frustration, repeated conflicts, and defensiveness. Marriages need a common operating language. "Sit down and learn each other's language before frustration turns your house into the Tower of Babel. Observe his method of communication and teach him yours."[4] In Marcus Buckingham's book *The One Thing You Need to Know,* he describes thriving marriages this way: "Each person believes his or her spouse to be better than the spouse actually believes him/herself to be. Or, you give me more credit for things than I give myself."[5] A goal in our marriage over many years has been to identify those things and verbalize them as much as possible to each other. We want to build each other up, affirm each other, and celebrate what we believe to be each other's strengths.

While training for the 2014 Chicago Marathon, my last mile included Lugers Hill. Runners in Holland know this to be a primary hill training route. On that day it was hot, and I was finishing a sixteen-mile run and could barely make it halfway up. My good friend Dan Broekhuizen must have seen me struggle up the hill, and he came running out of his house with some cool, refreshing water. The next day he sent me this message: "When you know someone else's Kolbe, you can refresh them." Yes, in a battle to live, to thrive, to heal, we must refresh others. "A generous person will prosper; whoever refreshes others will himself be refreshed" (Proverbs 11:25). Awareness is the first step in healing or changing.

CHAPTER 21
WHO IS IN YOUR BOAT?

I was too heavy for her, and she was too light for me.
—Søren Kierkegaard

It is those we live with and love and should know who elude us.
—Norman Mclean

One of my all-time favorite novels is Yann Martel's *Life of Pi*. It is a story of a young man (Pi) who survives a harrowing shipwreck and months in a lifeboat with a large Bengal tiger named Richard Parker.

In the story, Piscine Molitor Patel, more commonly referred to as Pi, finds himself on a cargo ship headed for Canada as his family immigrates there after selling their zoo in India. A terrible storm envelops the ship, and Pi is thrown onto a lifeboat. When he finally awakens the next morning, he sees the carnage and all he is left with. On the lifeboat, his companions are now a badly injured zebra, a violent hyena, a motherly orangutan, and under the canvas of the boat lies the tiger named Richard Parker. Over time and dwindling resources, the hyena kills the wounded zebra and orangutan. A once dormant Richard Parker eventually kills the hyena for preservation purposes. This leaves Pi and Richard Parker alone in a lifeboat to survive the elements for months on end. The remainder of the book details their fight for survival adrift in the Pacific.[1]

Who is in your boat? Do you respect, trust, and believe in them? Are they there to help you get through the voyage and gather the necessary food, water, and provisions to survive the journey? Or, is every moment of your life consumed by how you will keep them at bay, how you will minimize the anger and the flare-ups, and how you will create an environment so the journey can be smooth and calm. Are you on alert twenty-four hours a day because out of nowhere, they will pounce on you and eat you alive? I believe most marriages have seasons like Pi and Richard Parker. How do we stay as far apart from each other as possible? What do I need to do just to tame the tiger? How do I keep the strife at bay? What is going to set off the next big argument?

While golfing together early in our marriage, we both were standing on the top of the hill on the number eight hole at Clearbrook Golf Club looking over the creek to the green about 150 yards away. Chris was not playing very well on that day and was verbally frustrated. Other things were going on in our world and in his life right then. His confidence was low; his respect for me and for others was at an all-time bottom. Frankly, he didn't care what he said, to whom he said it, and when he said it. I usually keep a lot of my feelings to myself, but something got into me, and I needed to state the truth. I said, "I love you, but I just don't like you right now."

"We all see the picket fences or the pretty facades, the two smiling parents, the healthy siblings, all that, and part of us gets that we have zero idea what's going on behind closed doors, that there is anger and abuse, shattered dreams and blown expectations," says novelist Harlan Coben.[2] "A man's enemies will be the members of his own household" (Matthew 10:36).

Have you ever been so angry at your husband that the last thing you want to do is pray for him? My journey of praying for Chris started in 1999 with *The Power of a Praying Wife,* by Stormie Omartian.[3] This was the foundation upon which I would build the ability to pray daily for Chris once we understood his diagnosis fully. Praying for Chris needed to start with me.

Omartian says, "If you are angry at your husband, tell God. Don't let it become a cancer that grows with each passing day." She offers this approach as a prayer. "Lord, nothing in me wants to pray for this man.

I confess my anger, hurt, unforgiveness, disappointment, resentment, and hardness of heart toward him. Forgive me and create in me a clean heart and right spirit before You. Give me a new, positive, joyful, loving, forgiving attitude toward him ... Give my husband a new wife, and let it be me."[4]

Dr. Emerson Eggerichs, in his book *Love and Respect*, states, "There is an enormous amount of contempt inside our marriages today. Contempt, perhaps is the most corrosive force in marriage."[5] Much of this contempt is born out of unmet expectations—stated or unstated. Marriages will often experience irreparable damage when our expectations of each other do not coincide with the reality of who each one of us is. All of us everywhere need to lose the weight of these unmet expectations. The problem with family is that they have expectations; the great thing about friends is that they have none.

It was September 1989. I call this a Big Life Day. We were standing outside of the walk-in closet of our new home—a home we had moved into just weeks before. We were having a very intense argument about the state of my closet. In Chris's mind's eye it was in extreme disarray. "Your closet is a mess. Here we have this beautiful new home, and you treat it like this! There are dry cleaner bags everywhere. Your shoes are in a pile. Look at my side. It's well taken care of. Everything is in its place. You just don't care," exclaimed Chris. I was heartbroken. I did care; I cared deeply. It felt like he had just put a jagged-edge knife through my heart and then turned and twisted it. My heart was sliced and chopped into pieces. Oh, we kissed and made up from this scene, but it would not be until a year later when I was sitting in front of Kathy Kolbe, and she was giving me a personal interpretation of my Kolbe Index results that I realized how true Chris's words were. As a 2 in Follow Thru, I prevented and resisted keeping things neat, tidy, and in place. I resisted completing one thing at a time. I had great difficulty keeping anything in perfect order. I didn't need it that way, and so I didn't put striving energy into those efforts. But Chris absolutely needed it. What crystallized in that moment was that I did not care about what was important to my husband. His words, "you just don't care" were born out of his own viewpoint. I did care, but now I could see that I did not demonstrate actions around those things that were vitally important to him. So, in his mind, I did not care, and he was absolutely right. In our home, we call it Before Kolbe and After Kolbe.

"You don't know who you are until you are in a relationship with someone else," says Margaret Wheatley. It's the dynamic of the duo that creates the combustion. Nothing could be truer.

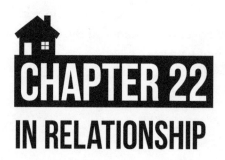

CHAPTER 22
IN RELATIONSHIP

Relationships have a uniqueness and a rhythm that confounds even the most brilliant of minds.
—*Michael Levins*

To love our neighbor as ourselves is such a truth for regulating human society, that by that alone one might determine all the cases in social morality.
—*John Locke*

King Solomon said in Proverbs 4:7, "Wisdom is supreme; therefore, get wisdom. Though it cost you all you have, get understanding." In other words, in all thy getting—get understanding! My belief is that right after prayer, God gave us Kolbe as a tool for getting the essential wisdom, understanding, and answers that we need to address the tough stuff of relationships, so we can make our lives work!

We need our relationships. And we need those relationships to work—especially in our marriages. There is probably no one person that you will spend more years of your life living with than your spouse. We fall in love; that's easy. The tough part is living together and making it work.

Psalm 133:1 says, "How good and pleasant it is when God's people live together in unity." Think of that picture, then think of your marriage. What are the things that you can think, do, or say that would make it pleasant for each other, that would make it good for each other, and would bring you together in unity? Along with that, consider how you would build each other up according to each one's specific needs. I have learned over the years that Chris *needs* things to be neat and tidy around our home. It's not something for him that would be nice to have, or that he selfishly *wants*. He *needs* it. It is an absolute necessity. There is a big difference between wanting it and needing it. Make it a priority to find out what your spouse needs. I'm serious here. Find out what your spouse truly needs in order to "be alive." The moment you discover that difference, your marriage will shift. Chris knows I have a need not to get boxed into rigid schedules. So, each of us is trying to provide the "air" for the other to be alive. But we are humans, and so we must work at making it work.

Years ago, I read *Growing Deeper in the Christian Life*, by Chuck Swindoll. In the book, Swindoll makes a case for the real consequences of sin. It goes like this. Adam and Eve sinned in the garden by disobeying God when they ate the fruit from the tree that God commanded them not to eat from. As a result, they sinned. Many believe the curse of sin to be that now we need to work, to toil through our lives. But Swindoll says no; the curse of sin is not work. Many of us love our work. Our work brings joy, engagement, fulfillment, and satisfaction. Swindoll says the real curse of sin is that we have to "deal with each other." The curse of sin is that we now must deal with those ugly differences that cause angst, strife, conflict, unmet expectations, hurt feelings, and sometimes even hatred.[1] I believe Swindoll's case for sin to be correct. But maybe the curse of sin does have to do with work—the need to *work at* dealing with each other. We need to work at being *in relationship* with each other. We need to put energy and effort into our most meaningful relationships. Whether those relationships are with family members, in the workplace, or at our churches and at our schools, we need to work at dealing with each other and meeting each other's needs so each of us can "be alive!"

(This is a personal note from Kathy Martin, our mother-in-law. No date—sometime before September 11, 2012)

Hi Mari & Chris—

We're excited about the Big Race, coming soon, and having you visit.

You will see changes in Jud—balance, walking, forgetfulness—fatigue, lack of appetite. He has not driven for weeks. On September 11 we both are having tests for understanding, etc. I'm very concerned. But I feel you have a right to know. He won't tell anyone on his own and I'm not telling him I wrote to the 2 of you just now!

There are times he is just fine & normal, and at other times very different. We try various foods, some are OK.

He is worried and so am I. So far, I'm a fairly good caregiver. I feel he is not in a bad situation, but he and I both lean toward downward at our age.

Don't worry more than you should, and I'll keep in touch with any changes or plans.

Blessings,
K

My mother-in-law was screaming out for help in this letter. She would pass away in May of the following year. Stay alert, and don't let yourself die of caregiving. Recognize when enough is enough. You must stay true to yourself, or you won't have the energy to give the proper care to your loved one.

And then, just when you think you can't do one more day, this arrives in the mail.

May 26, 2014

Happy Memorial Day, Mari—

Today's lull in the normal pace of life gives me a chance to write this letter which I've been meaning to write for several weeks. During Cindy's battle against breast cancer with chemo, radiation and two weddings (!?!) I learned what it means to be caregiver for those you love. I have admired from afar your extraordinary efforts and hope you call me if you ever just need to talk or unload. I would count it a privilege to join you on this journey. Do know that Cindy and I have both you and Chris in our prayers.

Wishing you God's peace,
Rob

Caregivers are seeking peace. They desperately need peace. Peace appears in the Bible 249 times. Many of those passages say, "Do you come in peace?" Or, "Go in peace." In Job's battles he cried out, "I have no peace, no quietness; I have no rest, but only turmoil" (Job 3:26). The word *peace* in Greek is *eireinei*. This eireinei has a wide semantic range including the notions of totality or completeness, success, fulfillment, wholeness, harmony, security, and well-being. Peace is associated with God's presence. Usually the term is used to refer to the experience of salvation that comes from God or the harmonious relationship between persons.[2] Peace is a mental attitude of tranquility in a relationship with God in the Christian way of life. It is a word which describes the result of a person's correct response to God's grace. Mitch Albom says, "because when the world quiets to the sound of your own breathing, we all want the same things: comfort, love, and a peaceful heart."[3]

Other caregivers know your anxieties. Like Rob, they have lived the life you are now living. Go to them for help. Receive some peace. Reach out to someone who can help. We reached out to hospice. Not because we thought Chris was ready to die but because we needed those around us who had traveled this journey time and time again. They knew the bends in the road. They knew where the path becomes dark and narrow. They knew the overhanging branches that would take us out from under our feet and drop us to the ground in an instant. They knew what we did not. At 3:00 a.m. if you cannot call when you are so anxious you can't live in your own skin anymore, call out to God. "The Lord gives strength to his people; the Lord blesses his people with peace" (Psalms 29:11).

Our pastor, Bill Boersma once gave a sermon on the Psalm 23. It was a time in our church when we were handed a worksheet as a guide for the sermon message. Bill's guide always included, "fill in the blank." It was that easy activity of fill in the blank that served as the foundation for me to memorize King David's honored words. These are words I have spoken over and over at 2:00 a.m., 3:00 a.m., and 4:00 a.m.

It says:

> The Lord *is* my shepherd, I shall not want. He makes me to lie down in green pastures; He leads me beside the still waters. He restores my soul; He leads me in the paths of righteousness For his name's sake. Yea, though I walk through the valley of the shadow of death, I will fear no evil; For you *are* with me; Your rod and Your staff, they comfort me. You prepare a table before me in the presence of my enemies; You anoint my head with oil; My cup runs over. Surely [SUrely, SURely, SUREly, SURELy, SURELY] goodness and mercy shall follow me All the days of my life; And I will dwell in the house of the Lord Forever. (Psalm 23:1–6 NKJV)

This might be a mixed version of different translations, but it is my version and the one I keep close to my heart so that I can call it forth ten, twenty, or thirty times during the day or night. It gives me peace. "And the peace of God, which surpasses all understanding, will guard your hearts and minds through Christ Jesus" (Philippians 4:7 NKJV).

Praying Psalm 23 for others:

Lord, You are her Shepherd. She knows that. Lord, You have presented Yourself to her, and she has experienced Your love and care. Help her to remember that. Help her to remember all those times and take comfort and trust You now in all things. Help her to trust You with her very life. You have provided for her, and she is grateful for the bounty that You have given to her throughout her life.

Help her now to experience sweet sleep, thinking only of Your love and care for her. Help her get the deep sleep she needs to heal her of all her diseases. Lead her to calming sounds and quiet waters that help her focus on what is true, what is noble, what is right, what is pure, what is lovely, what is admirable, what is excellent and praiseworthy. Help her to think on these things.

Restore her soul. Fill her with peace, joy, love, and, above all, Your nearness. Help her draw near to You, for when she does, You will draw near to her.

Guide her today down the straight path to righteousness. Take away the mountains and the valleys so she can preserve her energy and use it wisely to get to the place where You want her to be. Help her to proclaim Your Glory throughout her journey and to others along the way.

Today she is scared and frightened for her health diagnosis. Take away her anxious thoughts. Remove her fear. Comfort her with Your Presence. Help her to feel Your Presence and Your peace enfold over every inch and every cell in her body.

You, Lord, have called her through demons and battles throughout her life. She has remained faithful to You. Remember her faithfulness today. Help her remember all the deeds and miracles You have performed already throughout her life. Help her to meditate on all those mighty works that came from Your hand for her and her household.

Anoint her today, Lord, with a healing balm. Heal her body, heal her mind, heal her soul. May she taste the goodness of You and feel Your Presence and Your overflowing love.

Forgive all her sins. Keep her in your house today, tomorrow, and for all the beautiful days to come that she will experience. Hear my prayer for Donna today. In Jesus's name I pray. Amen.

Husbands, in the same way be considerate as you live with your wives, and treat them with respect as the weaker partner and as heirs with you of the gracious gift of life, so that nothing will hinder your prayers. (1 Peter 3:7)

Chris and I needed to work together to get him well. As a caregiver, I could first and foremost create an environment that mirrored his innate needs, as well as do willingly (without bitterness or resentment) what he could not do for himself. We needed to compensate for each other's inability. We would put our individual talents into play to complement each other. It's about figuring it out. There's a new strength in town, and they call it: figured-it-out-ness. As I write this, I am thinking about celebrating the thirty-six years that Chris and I have been married. I am proud of our marriage. We have figured it out. It has taken energy and effort, and I am proud of that. We have had to "work at" dealing with each other. In the most recent years our marriage has focused on Colossians 4:6: "Let your conversation be always full of grace, seasoned with salt, so that you may know how to answer everyone."

T. D. Jakes, in his book *The Great Investment: Faith, Family and Finance* says, "Grace renews the heart and reconciles the troubles of a tortured spirit. It is kindness and forgiveness. It is the favor of God, and as He bestows it on us, we should in turn give it to those who need our compassion and love."[4]

Thomas Friedman interviewed the US surgeon general, Vivek Murthy, for his recent book, *Thanks for Being Late: An Optimist's Guide to Thriving in the Age of Accelerations*. Murthy states: "We have such a fascination with new medicines and new cures, but if you think about it, compassion and love are our oldest medicines and they have been around for a millennia. When you practice medicine, you learn very quickly how much they are a part of the healing process."[5]

CHAPTER 23
DO NOT DIE OF CAREGIVING

Make a difference today for someone who
is fighting for their tomorrow.
—Jim Kelly

Self-care is not selfish. You cannot serve from an empty vessel.
—Eleanor Brownn

Are some of us hardwired to be caregivers? The Myers-Briggs Type Indicator actually gives the title: The Caregiver to the ESFJ pattern. ESFJ stands for Extroverted/Sensing/Feeling/Judging. People with this natural approach take their responsibilities very seriously. They are dependable and value security and stability. They have a strong focus for the details of life. They see before others do what needs to be done and do whatever it takes to make sure that it gets done. They are warm and energetic and do not understand unkindness. They are giving people who get a lot of personal satisfaction from the happiness of others. They are very sensitive to others and freely give practical care.[1] This certainly seems to be at the heart and soul of those who desire to provide care to others.

Paul Elzinga, the retired principal of Elzinga & Volkers in Holland, Michigan, shared a story with me several years back. I wanted to pursue it more, so recently I asked Paul to share these details over a cup of coffee.

When Paul attended Michigan Tech in Houghton, Michigan, where he pursued an engineering degree, he saw an opportunity posted on the bulletin board in his dormitory that caught his eye. The wife of a retired professor diagnosed with MS was looking for some young men to help her with her husband's daily needs. She was looking for four men to split duties around the clock to care for him. In exchange, they would receive room and board. This intrigued Paul, as he had seen his grandmother and aunts take care of his father. Paul states: "I got this caretaking sense from observing how well they took care of my father. It made a big impression on me."

These young male students covered everything from getting him up, changing his clothes, feeding, toileting, and exercising him around the clock. This was not an easy duty in exchange for room and board. The retired professor was angry. But these young engineering students found some meaning in their work as they developed a motorized bed that could provide him some exercise.

Paul did this for one to two years, he recalls, when he was nineteen years old. Many years later, when his wife, Pat, received a diagnosis of colon cancer, he sensed that what he had learned from caregiving then would be necessary for him to provide to his wife. During this time, he recalls mostly how women from their church organized care for Pat. He called them, "church family rallies."

Paul and many others, including my own sister, feel that their life's purpose is to provide care to others. My sister, Monica Morris, says, "I was put on this earth to care for Edward." My brother-in-law suffered with Parkinson's disease for many years before passing away in 2017, a couple of months after Hurricane Harvey [2] came roaring through their community.

My style of caregiving is not to sit at the bedside. I am more focused on what needs to happen next. My time frame is "the here and the now." Did you feed yourself? Can I help you with that? What bills need to be paid? Who will take you to your chemo treatment on Wednesday? Did you take all the doses of your medication today?

Caregivers take care of your psyche. Do not die of caregiving. Ask for help. "The local church is the hope for the world," Bill Hybels has said. Paul Elzinga concurs. There are "church ladies" that are ready, willing, and able to rally around you and support not only the patient but, more importantly, the caregiver. Be kind. Be generous. Be present. Be silent. Be sincere.

The power of faith is really the power of purpose. There is no denying that faith plays a role in longevity. The faithful are on to something, in that they live longer and apparently happier lives, moment to moment. There is evidence that cancer progresses more slowly in people with friends than in people who feel lonely.[3]

Friends are an immense gift anytime but especially during an uncomfortable journey with cancer. Jay and Jeanne Lindell write: "Yet in the midst of these trials we have experienced God's grace through the love, care and assistance of the community of faith that surrounds us—friends who are comfortable walking with us on this difficult journey. We never would have chosen this journey we have, but we have never been alone in it."

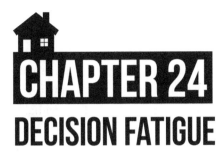

CHAPTER 24
DECISION FATIGUE

We are what we repeatedly do. Excellence then, is not an act, but a habit.
—*Aristotle*

There's nothing you can't do if you get the habits right.
—*Charles Duhigg*

It virtually became a Friday afternoon routine. When you are sick, there are going to be bills. And lots of them. I had created a habit on Friday afternoons to head over to the office of our health insurance provider with our mountain of bills. Each week we would receive the reports from the various procedures, office visits, hospital stays, and tests that Chris needed. During the week, I'd gather all these together. There were bills for the chemotherapy, the radiation treatments, the doctor consultations, the PET scans, the nutrition, the ER visits, and the hospital stays. Life for me in March was overwhelming figuring out what would be the amount we must pay. The radiation alone was a $75 copay per visit. It doesn't take long to multiply that times thirty-nine, and with that treatment approach alone, our responsibility was close to $3,000. That was only one of the many procedures he was prescribed.

"Decision making depletes your willpower, and once your willpower is depleted, you're less able to make decisions ... the depleted state makes people look for ways to postpone or evade decisions," says John Tierney, author of *Willpower*. "Orderly habits can actually improve self-control in the long run by triggering automatic mental processes that don't require much energy."[1] Decision fatigue affects us all. By creating a habit to do something, we use less willpower. We have a limited amount of self-control strength, and as we exert it, we exhaust it. Habits make change possible by freeing us from decision-making and from using self-control. Committing the more mundane parts of our lives to habit and routine frees up RAM for the things that matter most. If we have created the habit, then we won't need to use self-control or willpower. For example, I run three days each week. It's always three—but not the same three.

This is the system that I have put into place. I don't have to get motivated because it's just part of the routine. If I can stick to my system, then I won't need to muster up the motivation. Doing something requires willpower. It takes energy to go from desire to action. Many of us put our precious mental energy into thinking about doing something, or wanting to do something, instead of just doing it. Having a system brings clarity. When our life patterns are disrupted, and our lives are in flux, we get ill. "What most people don't realize is that your habits don't follow your ambition, they follow your system."[2]

It is tiring to decide. Kolbe helps us recognize the decisions that will be exhausting for us but that seem so easy and obvious to others. We have self-control in some ways but not in others. Through Kolbe, you can be more aware of those actions that you will procrastinate because you now understand that innately you are avoiding, putting off, resisting, or preventing. This is also where you experience fear, fatigue, and frustration.[3] What is your friction or pain point? It is where you have less mental energy. Recognize it. Identify it. Name it. With this type of self-awareness, we can more easily figure out how to minimize stress and be more purposeful.

My trip to Priority Health on Friday afternoons saved me from decision fatigue. I could tap into the expert there who would sift through the complexities of all the statements that had accumulated that week. My 4 in Fact Finder needed someone I could rely on who could dig, delve, and investigate each one of the services and give me peace of mind that I was paying only what was necessary. Part of the habit of going there was taking the checkbook along so I would write out the checks and get those services paid for. My innate tendency, driven by the 2 in Follow Thru, is to hold off and not bring closure. I invariably believe a better or easier option will come along. Together, we developed a treasure of trust during those weeks we met, as many times she would say, "Don't pay that bill yet. Don't pay that bill, we are having problems with that vendor right now. I'll look into it for you."

CHAPTER 25
THIS COULD GO EITHER WAY

We forget that the water cycle and the life cycle are one.
—*Jacques Yves Cousteau*

And, above all, watch with glittering eyes the whole world around you because the greatest secrets are always hidden in the most unlikely places.
—*Roald Dahl*

Tulip Time in Holland, Michigan, is a jam-packed week of tulips, shows, tulips, Dutch Dancers, geedunk trucks, stomachaches from the street food, fireworks, tulips, parades, shows, more parades. And did I mention, five million tulips? It is a spectacular week each year when our town gets to strut its stuff for over five hundred thousand guests who want to anticipate the perfect time for viewing the many varieties and colors of tulips that are bursting forth along the main thoroughfares, as well as quiet neighborhoods throughout the city. It is the largest tulip festival in the United States. The week of festivities kicks off with the Tulip Time Run. There are two runs. A 5K and a 10K are available to run. What's cool is you can run both for the price of one. That was what I had registered for several months earlier.[1]

We now were about eight weeks posttreatment, yet Chris was not improving. He was uncomfortable and had no energy to manage his daily routine—meaning, he wasn't getting dressed in the morning. His appearance is of utmost importance to him. He is perfectly organized and holds himself to that standard with his hair, clothes, and personal look. I felt guilty leaving, but he insisted I go. He was still planning to get to Christ Memorial Church's parking lot to see me as I ran by. We calculated the time and double-checked the meet up spot. I'd be gone at most two hours, so I left anticipating the crowds, the energy, and the overall jubilation of the day.

The 10K route was the one Chris would be on. It's a route I had run several times during training leading up to the race. One quarter mile from our home, and I was on the route. It winds through South Shore Drive and into homey neighborhoods on the south side of our town before ending on Washington Boulevard and a final surge up Twelfth Street. Both are boulevards with multiple layers of tulips bursting out in full color for several blocks.

I am running up Plasman Avenue directly headed to Twenty-Fourth Street where the route turns east. At that turn is the driveway headed into Christ Memorial Church. That's where he said to look for him. I could see his car parked right there. He made the effort to get dressed and drive the short distance to the parking lot. As I get closer, I wondered who the man was standing next to, and hanging on to, the car door. *That man is not Chris. Is this someone's ninety-year-old grandfather?* This man looked tiny, as if he was withering away to nothing. But this man had on a golf hat that I knew to be Chris's, so it had to be him. It was one our son had given him from the Ryder Cup held at the Medinah Golf Club in Chicago just two years earlier. The cap was too big. It covered his ears. He was literally grasping onto the car door to keep his balance. I ran up to him, held his face and kissed him, and thanked him for coming. He had worked incredibly hard just to get to that very spot. Both of us were captured by the moment.

I should have stopped right then. But I kept going. I was out to lunch.

CHAPTER 26
TROUBLING SYMPTOMS

I have told you these things, so that in me you may
have peace. In this world you will have trouble.
But take heart! I have overcome the world.
—John 16:33

Trouble is here. It is for a purpose. Use it for
the purpose for which it was intended—to help
you grow. Thank God for your troubles.
—Norman Vincent Peale

That moment. That kiss. The look we gave to each other said it all.
Chris was dying. I knew it, and what was harder to handle is that
he knew it too. There were some troubling symptoms we needed to
confront with each other. He continued to lose weight by the day.
He had zero energy to feed and dress himself. And now, there was
something else. The left side of his neck showed signs of a protruding
growth of some sort. Neither of us wanted to mention it or acknowledge
it. But it was there and getting larger as each of us refused to state the
obvious.

Maybe it was how much I was shocked at his appearance as I ran
toward him. So often you are right in the battle, and you simply can't
see what's real. What was real is that Chris was not bouncing back after

treatments as the doctors indicated. Chris was heading into a death spiral. What could change the trajectory of our despair?

Early on, Dr. Edlund said, "We will take you to the doorstep of death and then bring you back again." How do you know which doorstep that is? Is it marked? Is there some kind of indicator that says, "Yes, this is the one: go no further?" I continued to hear the words *you are not a doctor*, which did give me peace that someone else was in charge of the specific doorstep.

On his own, could he continue to fight the overwhelming desire to quit when the air he was breathing right now was really thin? He was freezing to death from the inside out. I was shocked at how much change had occurred right under my own eyes, and I failed to see the progression taking place. Could he harness the little will he had to fight for his life today? This is the Big Life Day. It is today. Off to the emergency room we went.

CHAPTER 27
WORDS AND ACTIONS REALLY MATTER

Truth without love is brutality. Love
without truth is hypocrisy.
—H. H. Charles

The truth does not need to be defended.
—Elizabeth Kubler-Ross

After all the preliminary screening was done in the emergency room, Chris was given an actual hospital room. With that, we knew for sure he would stay the night there. I gladly was ready for others to take the lead, carry the load, and shoulder the responsibility. Some good friends and neighbors were at the hospital visiting other people and stopped by the room to check in with us. About this time an aide came in and put up the guardrails on Chris's bed. She also started fitting him with what looked like combatant gear. It seemed very strange at the time and was truly alarming, especially with guests in the room observing these preparations. The gear was white and gave the impression he was ready to be announced for the next karate match. Everything was there except for the colored belt. All this was taking place while our friends tried to carry on a casual conversation.

It became too unnerving for me, and so I questioned the aide. "What is this for? Why are the guardrails up? What are those things you are putting on his arms?"

She was only doing her job. She was carrying out the orders that someone else told her. But what were those orders and why these preparations? I didn't want to appear confrontational, but this was over the line in my estimation. When I questioned her, she simply said, "I'll have to get someone else to share that with you."

We were certainly on edge that day. Both of us sensed that Chris was losing his life. Now these preparations were being made. What did all this mean? Fairly soon a nurse came in to give us the details. Here's what was happening. Chris's sodium levels in the blood work came back extremely low. When this occurs, the patient can feel tired, confused, and experience a loss of energy. There is also the chance they can become irritable and disoriented. Sometimes they can go into a coma and have convulsions. There can also be other neurological manifestations. What happened to us on that day was that the cart came before the horse. Timing is everything.

The nurse got hung up on some other project and lost sight of the fact that the aide was going to do her work. We were trapped in a time warp where everything was unraveling. It is so essential for communication to be provided in the proper sequence.

I was still recovering from the scare of this news and the unfolding of the preparations prior to the proper information relay when I headed down the hallway to the bathroom. A conversation was happening between two EMT technicians. It went something like this:

"We are preparing to transport the patient in room 442 to St. Mary's. He has a tumor growing uncontrollably on the side of his neck."

All I heard was uncontrollably. I was stopped in my tracks. Low sodium levels. Hmm. What else don't we know? What is being withheld from us? He's being transported? He won't be staying the night? Why won't they talk straight? Who is in charge here? And get me to that person *now*.

I now know that cancer doesn't grow uncontrollably. It grows slowly. But on that day, I did not know that. My world was flat out falling apart. Chris was transported to St. Mary's Hospital, where his oncologist could begin understanding the situation and prescribing the necessary steps for dealing with these two new side effects. The low sodium apparently was the underlying symptom of how I saw the man I loved grasping the side of the car door earlier that day at our meetup point. The neck tumor appearance may just have been the ticket to get us to the hospital and get Chris some proper treatment so he could come back to life. Praise the Lord, and we are thankful for the uncontrollable growth on the side of his neck.

What we learned through the course of the next two days was that the neck growth was most possibly due to a large amount of sloughing of membrane and neck tissue from a massive coughing spell that Chris had a few weeks earlier. He most likely had a hernia. But we weren't going to leave it there. He would head back to Ann Arbor to Dr. Prince and his team for a biopsy due to these troubling symptoms and suspicious spots.

CHAPTER 28
WORDS THAT ENCOURAGE

Applause is the spur of noble minds,
the end and aim of weak ones.
—Edmund Burke

The more you focus on words that uplift you, the more
you embody the ideas contained in those words.
—Oprah Winfrey

How can we be encouraging to others? Think before we speak. Think about how our words will be heard, received, and understood. Had the EMT known the woman headed down the hall to the restroom was the wife of the patient with the tumor growing uncontrollably on the side of his neck, I'm sure he would not have made those comments. Or the comment, "My, how your mother has aged," that I heard spoken to the son whose mother had just died of lung cancer.

Now we are in the examining room with Dr. Prince and his team of young residents prior to the scheduled biopsy. The radiation treatments have closed Chris's jaw, and he is only able to open his mouth about three-fourths of an inch. One of the residents noticed this and said, "We'll never be able to get in there."

Dr. Prince looked over at Chris and chimed right in without a hitch or a beat or a pause, "Piece of cake."

CHAPTER 29

JUST BETWEEN YOU AND ME

Wise men talk because they have something to say; fools because they have to say something.
—*Plato*

Maturity means that everything you think doesn't need to be said.
—*T. D. Jakes*

Whether it is his natural gift, or it has been developed through his radio work, Chris has commentary. I have told him many times he was just ahead of the whole ESPN curve. When we watch a sports event together on TV, he will provide the color commentary after the play. Sometimes right during the play he'll make a comment, and it's almost uncanny that the announcer will say exactly what he just said to me. When this happens, it is fun to hear, and I'll stoke the fire. There are other times when I can take it or leave it. And there are definitely times when it becomes irritating, even annoying, and I just need silence.

A person, when given the power to use his or her voice, discovers well on what topics to silence that voice. Not every thought needs to be spoken. If you are suffocating because you feel that no one is listening to you or that you do not matter, it may be that you have yet to discover when your silence is, in truth, your power. "Teach me, and I will be quiet; show me where I have been wrong. How painful are honest words!" (Job 6:24–25).

I run to hear what the Lord is trying to teach me. One message was *It's just between you and me.* What I take away from that is, *There are things you just keep to yourself. Take up your drama and complaints with me. I can handle everything. Others don't need to know that you feel this is unfair. Just tell me. Guard your lips to guard your life.* And so, I long to hear these messages, but I must be silent.

In the October 11 devotional—"After God's Silence—What?"— from Oswald Chambers's book *My Utmost for His Highest,* Chambers says,

> Has God trusted you with a silence? … God's silences are His answers … His silence is the sign that He is bringing you into a marvelous understanding of Himself … If God has given you a silence, praise Him.[1]

I learned a lot about silence during June 2014. Chris was not improving. He was still sleeping all the time. We'd already had one biopsy to identify if there were still cancerous cells in his throat. Dr. Gribben said very matter-of-factly, "This could go either way." It was at lunch one day with my associate, Monica Gravenhof, and her parents that the cold reality began to set in—he may not make it.

They were there letting me share aloud what was locked away in my heart. We have come to a time when *this could go either way.* In their silence, they were letting me verbalize Chris's status so the weight of the circumstances would begin to lose its controlling power.

I'll be honest. This was the time I thought about Chris's funeral and what I would say. Chris has a great sense of humor, and I wanted people to know that. I thought about it for a few days and realized that I needed to start with his commentary. There will be a couple of days when I will welcome the silence and even enjoy it. But then, I will not only want the commentary but need it from him. Because that's him, and it's all of him that I love.

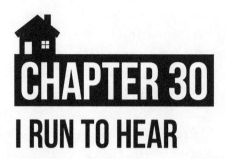

CHAPTER 30

I RUN TO HEAR

In whom are hidden all the treasures of wisdom and knowledge.
—*Colossians 2:3*

When you are in the dark, listen, and God
will give you a very precious message.
—*Oswald Chambers*

Several years after my father battled colon cancer, he shared with me during that time of his life that he was never closer to the Lord. But he also said, "I don't ever want to have to go through the same ravage of my body to get that close to God. Mari, apart from dying, try to find a time while you are yet living to hear what God wants you to know."

I run to help me keep a clear mind and a sound mind amid so much uncertainty. While on my training runs, I begin to get a glimmer of what I think the Lord wants to tell me through the Holy Spirit. Each of the eight marathons I have run has brought me an incredible message and a blanket of peace. During my times alone, those miles allow me to focus on the One who can handle every one of the problems I might have. After I run, my hopes and dreams seem all that much more plausible. Jesus, my family, and running—they lift me up when the world wants to drag me down.

For me, it's not about the marathon. It's about practicing the necessary discipline for sixteen weeks that says I am worthy to even be standing in the start gate.

And so, I run to hear. Many long hours alone, mostly in the dim light of dawn. In a more exhausted state, sometimes while training, but oftentimes during the race, I will hear very personalized whispers. Maybe it's the uninterrupted time alone. Maybe it's the depleted physical state. Maybe it's the cry for help. Maybe it's for real. I believe they are real. I know they are real. These are messages that God wants me to hear, while I am yet living.

The first one was very soft—*Choose the better thing. That will make all the difference in the world.* The next one was loud and long—*My child, I love you and have mercy on you; I give you my grace and my guidance, now go and do likewise.* Each one comes at a special time in my life when I am struggling with something such as health, finances, or relationships. These are the Big Three. Imagine heading out for a training run and bam, out of the clear, comes a bullet of wisdom that is totally meant for you. It is an elixir. It is also addicting. Once you hear it, you clamor for more.

All the messages I have heard are close to my heart. I have each of them memorized with the place where the experience happened. I can draw from each one when clouds get dark and life isn't going well. None seems to be more important than another. It's like a package deal. Each is just perfect, at just the right time. Together, they are totally remarkable. Simple, yet powerful, and utterly mind blowing.

Undoubtedly, the marathon that has special meaning to me is the one I ran in Green Bay in 2010. The spectators there put a whole new perspective on "cheering the runners on." The following describes the experience I believe would lift you up and carry you through the months—maybe years—of treatment and recovery that is required to Come Home Alive.

It starts at 1265 Lombardi Avenue. People in Wisconsin know this address well. It is Packer Stadium. You literally get to go inside the stadium and hang out prior to the race. You can browse around and look at memorabilia or head up to the gift shop and peer in to see what extra gear you might need or want to buy to remember the experience. And best of all, you can go to a real bathroom. You are not limited to a portable john experience, not at the start of the race. You feel comfortable—right at home.

With that available, the wait time doesn't feel awkward; you can head out to the start line when you feel ready, as it's just out the doors of the stadium and down a few stairs to the street. There are hardly any prerace jitters this way. Then the gun goes off, and you are on your way. Sweet. There is no awkward wait.

The best part of the Green Bay Marathon is the way the spectators cheer you on. They are not standing on the edge of the street six people deep like Chicago. They are literally in their driveway, on chaise lounges with blankets around them, holding their massive size coffees, and taking in the view. Behind them is what I would describe as a "honking size" grill, already stoked, with smoke rising and the smell of brats, hot dogs, and hamburgers. The portable stereo is blasting some upbeat tune that gives you a pep in your step. And this goes on, driveway after driveway after driveway. It almost says, "We're not making a big deal out of this; we want to be there for you, but life goes on, grab a brat!"

The beauty of Green Bay is that the first half of the route mostly flows through regular streets and neighborhoods. Spectators are talking to each other, laughing, holding babies, and drinking coffee, glad to be in their driveway and not out on the road with us. Then there is a transition to a more industrial and commercial area before heading across the bridge over the Fox River to downtown De Pere. There you catch a river trail all the way north to downtown Green Bay.

On the river trail, families have made a special effort to get there. They parked their cars, hauled out the strollers or bikes or whatever will keep the youngsters occupied, and walked down to the trail to see their friend, aunt, uncle, mom, or dad run by. Their signs are raised high. "Aunt Sara, look, here we are. We made this sign for you. RUN REALLY FAST AUNT SARA." Families on the right; nature on the left.

We transition back through downtown Green Bay and head south to Lambeau Field. Yes, Lambeau Field is the finish line. I can just hear Chris Berman of ESPN: "the frozen tundra of Lambeau Field." On this day, the tundra is not frozen. It is pristine. Not a blade of grass is out of place. The field is immaculate. In Wisconsin, it is revered.

There is not a more fitting finish to a marathon than in Green Bay. You are steered toward a tunnel that takes you inside the stadium. You look straight up into the jumbotron and hear Queen's "We are the Champions"[1] blasting loudly throughout the stadium. You see the stadium in all its glory with the thousands of seats that would be filled to overflowing on a fall Sunday. You are no longer tired. The journey has not worn you out. You know the finish is just on the other side of the track around the field, and out into the bright daylight again. But you want to linger. You are not sprinting through this moment. You want to savor these few last steps, strides, even. You want to remember this time and this place. You are proud of the journey and how far you have come. You know you can cross the finish line now. You want to ponder awhile on the entire experience. You want to reflect on the whisper: *Send her My love.* It came at such a quiet moment. Running over the bridge into De Pere. You have been there and now you are back. *Attraversiamo*—a beautiful, graceful Italian word for crossover. You have been across the river, and now you have come home to the cheers, the applause, the hearty smiles, and welcomes. You are someone. You are real. You will not be forgotten. You were away, but now you are back.

"4:24. Mom, you had a 4:24 today," said Ara as we crossed the finish line on that day in Chicago back in 2006. Our hands were clasped together, raised high over our heads.

"4:24? Are you crazy? No, I didn't. Not on your life," I responded.

"Yes, Mom, you did. You trained well. You should have left me back there," he said.

"That's not what we agreed to. We agreed to run together, stay together, and finish together. You would have done the same for me. You helped me do this. We agreed to stay together. And we did, to the very end," I said.

"Not discounting, you still had a 4:24 in you today, know that," Ara said, looking me squarely in the eyes. *Choose the better thing. That will make all the difference in the world.*

As you fight this battle, what do you have in you? What'd ya got? I like to think of the marathons I've run like this:

- The first one tells you what you got (4:24, huh?).
- The second one puts you in your place.
- The third one is the charm (4:22:21).
- The fourth one confirms that the third one isn't a fluke (4:22:54).

What do you got? Only we can know what is inside us. Only Chris would be the one to determine the kind of fight he had. How would he stay motivated to fight the overwhelming desire to quit? How could he harness his will to punch through from the doorstep of death to push past the thin air, when he had no desire to sustain himself and make it back to the land of the living.

The following is a combination of all the messages in the form of a prayer I use for assurance:

> Choose the better thing today. That will make all the difference in the world. My child, I love you, and I have mercy on you. I give you My grace and My guidance; now go and do likewise. Hold fast to the Word of Life. When you do, your doubts and fears will vanish. I send you My love. I wait for you, Oh Lord, and in Your Word I put my hope. My love pours over you as you wait. Get up—you are here to bring life and growth to others. This is a gift; be faithful. Turn someone else's water into wine. Guard your lips to guard your life. Take up your complaints and drama with Me. It's just between you and Me. Join with Me, Stay with Me, have peace with Me. I am calling you to tell somebody something that will save their life. Take every step in obedience to Me, and you will see My glory. You are a bright and shining star. Remember, you can do all things through Christ who strengthens you. He will keep you strong to the end.

I am running again. Maybe not marathons, but Turkey Trots and Tulip Time Runs—5 and 10Ks. I'm back out on the streets of my new neighborhood, looking to connect with specific homes and the people inside. On one particular street, I have picked out six homes in a stretch. Home #1 is all brick and very stately. I often notice the two white vehicles in the driveway. Home #3 has a warm and welcoming front porch with two Adirondack chairs, just meant for taking it easy. There are small white lights strung from the ceiling. These are always lit, no matter the time of day. Home #6 sports the American flag flying proudly in the wind. They are just six random homes I picked out one morning. Why six? Statistics show that one in every three females will get cancer in her lifetime. Home one and four. One in every two males will be diagnosed with cancer in his lifetime.[2] Homes one, three, and five. As I run by these six homes I think, yes, no, yes, yes, yes, no. I think a lot about Home #1. It is the stately brick one. From the outside everything is solid. But what's going on inside that home if this is the one where both a male and female have been diagnosed with cancer? How are they doing? Who is helping them? Did this happen at the same time? I pray over these six homes when I run by. I pray for what is already happening, and what each of them might soon discover.

CHAPTER 31
WHAT I HAVE LEARNED ABOUT CANCER

The more I read, the more I acquire, the more certain I am that I know nothing.
—*Voltaire*

Frequent visits to doctors are a potentially hazardous activity to engage in.
—*Steven Magee*

Cancer is a disease of the old. Many people don't get cancer because they die before they get old. I've learned that certain cancers grow slowly. You don't wake up one day with a tumor on the side of your throat. Things have been moving and changing for perhaps decades. There are signs that precancerous cells already exist. We all need to be alert to these signs and signals. We certainly hope the doctors that we trust with our health care will see them ahead of time and order the right tests and procedures for earlier detection.

I have learned that doctors are treating the disease but are not giving patients and their families a road map to navigate the terrain they will be on. In a *View from the Front Line*, Maggie Jencks describes her experience likened to being shoved out of a "Jumbo Jet" with a parachute into a foreign landscape, but with no map: You descend. You hit ground ... but where is the enemy? What is the enemy? What is it up to? No road. No compass. No map. No training. Is there something you should know and don't?[1]

These might be some of the questions we need answered before we get that shove. If I land alive, what then? Do I need to turn right or left? How far is the closest town? Will there be provisions when I get there? Can I get there by foot, or will I need to hitch a ride? Who is on the road with me, and can I trust them? What country am I in? What language do they speak? My hope is that for those that have a similar diagnosis as Chris's, you understand what will happen when you hit the ground.

I've learned that our lifestyle choices can absolutely contribute to higher risks for a cancer diagnosis. What we eat, drink, and do to our bodies elevates the risk for developing cancer during our lifetimes. I have learned there are over one hundred types of cancer. I have learned that someone can have more than one type of cancer at the same time. I have learned that a virus may cause cancer. I have learned not to say cancer free, as cancer can recur. In the end, cancer is a cruel disease.

I have learned that we have not curbed the number of cancer diagnoses. The rates for people who will be diagnosed with cancer continue to increase.[2] Even with the billions of dollars that have been allocated toward research, there is yet to be found a universal cure. But people are surviving and living through this diagnosis. Treatments are constantly improving. In the United States, an estimated 15.5 million people with a history of cancer were living as of January 1, 2016.[3] This is all very encouraging.

I've learned that if there are screening tests for any type of cancer, get in line. Do it. You will not die of a colonoscopy. You can survive a gallon of collate. You can manage an evening in your bedroom with a good book next to the toilet. Get screened as often as your medical plan will allow. Get a mammogram every year if you can. Do breast self-examinations. Get a PAP smear routinely according to plan guidelines. The PAP smear is not to find cancer, but to identify signs that cells could turn into cancer.[4] A Mayo Clinic study in 2019 showed that less than two-thirds of women ages thirty to sixty-five are current on cervical cancer screenings.[5] These are not difficult procedures to endure. Do not let any of these opportunities to screen go by. Find out any and all screening tests that are approved by your medical plan. Challenge your doctor to get those scheduled. Screening leads to detection of unusual cell growth earlier. Screening can potentially identify precancerous growth. It might ensure you don't hear T4 N2b M0.

I've learned that diabetes and cancer have similarities. "Both diabetes and cancer are related to obesity, inflammation and increased blood sugar."[6] "One trait of cancer cells is that they are adept at absorbing glucose from the blood with no need for insulin. Since cancer runs on glucose, high blood glucose levels may help fuel the growth of cancer cells."[7] I learned that the doctors don't tell you all this. I certainly don't know why. There is much research to show that people with diabetes have an increased risk of dying from cancer, compared to those without the disease.[8]

If your loved one has type 2 diabetes, then realize that certain cancer medications can worsen diabetes complications. Elevated blood sugars make tolerating cancer treatment more difficult. You must keep blood sugar levels in target ranges to prevent treatment interruptions, infection, and weight loss. Stay well hydrated, and don't skip meals. Go into the treatment phase with your eyes wide open. Chemotherapy can worsen blood glucose levels. Work with your doctor in advance to devise a plan that will address and even prevent these side effects.[9]

Our issue was dehydration. Dehydration delays treatment. When dehydration sets in, the imbalance can lead to confusion, dizziness, weakness, and ultimately fainting, as with Chris. Since Chris was only getting his liquids through the feeding tube, I was not sure how much or how little he was getting. If he didn't feel like setting up the science lab, he didn't. If his stomach wouldn't accept the fluid, he quit. It proved to be a big problem—possibly his biggest problem during the treatment phase.

I have learned there are many distinguished books to read, if you want to immerse yourself in greater awareness. Not everyone who encounters cancer in their world has read, or even would want to read, the *Emperor of all Maladies, A Biography of Cancer*, by Siddhartha Mukherjee. Given our experience, I wanted to know more and felt this could fill in some missing pieces. It also wasn't learning about cancer on the internet. It tells the history of cancer treatment and research up to our present age.[10] I found it to be not only informative about cancer diagnosis and treatment, but also chock-full of personal, oftentimes heartbreaking and intimate, stories of many individuals and their unique journey. It provided me with some answers but left me asking many more questions. The biggest question: Why, with all the research and billions of dollars spent, are we continuing to see cancer diagnosis going up?

But I've also learned that cancer is not a death sentence; it is just a word. Years ago, when people received a cancer diagnosis, we stood back. We didn't want to touch them. We thought it would jump onto us. We'd get it too.[11] Cancer patients need our touch. They need us to reach out and hold them close. Cancer is not contagious, but it can be hereditary. Make good lifestyle choices.

I have just finished reading a marvelous novel by Peggy Hesketh, *Telling the Bees*.[12] It left me wanting more of her words and her style. I found out this was her only novel. She had passed away at the young age of sixty-four. I do not know if she died of cancer. I do know from her obituary that she had breast cancer at some point in her lifetime. I was sad—sad for her family and sad for her readers, like me, who wanted more. When cancer takes someone's life, we lose out. There will be no more books, no more dances, no more shows, no more songs, no more news stories or sportscasts, no more performances, no more movies, no more experiences. But we will have the memories of people like: Peter Jennings, Patrick Swayze, Farrah Fawcett, George Harrison, Ingrid Bergman, Stuart Scott, Randy Pausch, Humphrey Bogart, Gilda Radner, and Paul Newman.

Ultimately the most indelible and lasting impression I have come to understand is that cancer is unique to each person and to each situation. It is an N-of-1. The future of cancer treatment lies in providing patients with an ever-greater level of personalization.[13] We must look closer at the individual experience with the cure. That will be the new breakthrough: *Listen to the unheard, and see the invisible.*

Enter his gates with thanksgiving and his courts with praise; give thanks to him and praise his name.

Psalm 100:4

PART 6

BE GRATEFUL AND THANKFUL

CHAPTER 32
BE GRATEFUL AND THANKFUL

Prayer and praise are the oars by which a man may row
his boat into the deep waters of the knowledge of Christ.
—*Charles Spurgeon*

O Lord that lends me life, lend me a
heart replete with thankfulness.
—*William Shakespeare*

Over the years, our work has taken us to destinations we would not normally have the chance to see. One engagement with the Rescue Mission of Los Angeles took place at a convent overlooking the Pacific Ocean in Malibu, California. It was breathtaking.

We have traveled the roads from Holland to Detroit so often I think the car was autonomous, even without the technology we have today. We have traveled to England, Connecticut, Georgia, Florida, New York, New Jersey, South Carolina, and many other states across the nation, especially in the Midwest. One engagement with Audi of Canada brought us to Toronto to focus on creating a service approach that was distinctive and would set them apart from their competition. We were checked into one of the finest hotels in the Yorkville area. However, during the night, all we could hear was what we determined to be street thugs and hooligans. Their shrill voices dominated the darkness. Their screams were loud and piercing through the night, reminding me of ceremonies with war chants. We did finally get some rest and were up early for a very full day with the most elite Audi dealership in downtown Toronto. Our car was parked in the hotel parking lot, four stories down.

What a shock to arrive at the car and have the driver-side window bashed in and totally demolished, cracked to pieces. We had obviously been vandalized and robbed. We looked around tentatively, at first, hoping to avoid any sharp pieces of glass that might cut our skin. Shards of glass were everywhere. How could this have happened? Where was the security? After a quick perusal of the interior, we determined that Chris's briefcase was probably the only thing that was missing. The Garmin we used for navigation was still tucked away under the passenger seat in the front. Luckily, we had not left any other valuables that we could recall in the car. We had no time to feel sorry for ourselves. We needed to be off so we could arrive on time and be prepared to provide the training and coaching the team was looking forward to.

How convenient that we were working with a car dealership. Our car would need some repairs, certainly, and here we were with the Garmin still in our possession, and the address where friends and future friends would welcome us, assure our safety, and fix our car. How convenient was that. The drive to the dealership included something we didn't need right then—rain. Pouring rain. Hard, driving, pelting, windy, gusty raindrops were falling everywhere inside the car. On us, on the seats, on our presentation. But we were safe. We were not harmed. How will we give the proper thanks for that?

While in Toronto I also happened to be reading Ann Voskamp's *One Thousand Gifts*. It is one of my absolute treasures and was given to me by my sister-in-law. It is a practical guide to living a life of joy and includes ways to wake up to God's everyday blessings. "Is the height of my (*chara*) joy dependent on the depths of my (*eucharisteo*) thanks?" The word eucharisteo came to mind through the driving wind and rain. "The greatest thing is to give thanks for everything. He who has learned this knows what it means to live ... He has penetrated the whole mystery of life: giving thanks for everything."[1]

Dear Lord, thank you for leaving the Garmin. Thank you that we have the right address. Thank you that the tires were not ruptured. Thank you that we could get into the car. Thank you that it works. Thank you that we know where to go. Thank you for people who will welcome us and put our fears to rest.

I continued to give thanks through the driving rain, through the unfamiliar route, and through the uncertainty of how the day would unfold. Voskamp's salient words penetrated my mind: "What precedes the miracle is thanksgiving, eucharisteo."[2]

We believed that God would heal Chris, but we needed to be a part of the equation. During our routine of praying together each morning, we gave thanks for each small yet potentially significant step in the healing process.

We gave thanks for our doctors. We gave thanks for the research and the treatment plan. We gave thanks for Todd, our very attentive technician at the Lemmon Holton Cancer Facility. We gave thanks for the nurses and aides that attended to Chris in the hospital. We gave thanks for Bill Boersma, our pastor who always arrived at just the right time, had the most concise words for the moment, and left when there was nothing more he could do. We gave thanks for Monica, back in the office, who was managing all the pieces and literally holding the business together.

We gave thanks for cards that arrived in the mail. We gave thanks for friends that arrived with food for the day and food for the week. We gave thanks for all those who drove Chris to his treatment. We gave thanks that we were figuring out the feeding tube, so Chris could get the calories and the liquids that were so essential for his healing.

We gave thanks for the service we received at Priority Health helping to sort out the mountain of bills that would be our responsibility. We gave thanks that we had built up enough of a balance in our health saving account so we could pay the bills we needed to that month. We gave thanks for our family and their prayers, their concern, and their questions. We gave thanks that Chris was sleeping twenty hours a day. Whatever we experienced, we found some way to see it as an essential part of the journey and to express eucharisteo.

I reviewed my Prayer Focus, which included: give thanks for answers that are already under way, even though you haven't seen any outward, visible signs. This reminds me of the story of the ten lepers in the book of Luke. During one of Jesus's travels, His final trip to Jerusalem, in fact, He encountered ten leprous men. The lepers didn't need to say, "Heal us of our leprosy!" All they needed to do was cry out, "Jesus, Master, have pity on us!" (Luke 17:13). When Jesus saw their disease, He already knew what their need was. "'Go, show yourselves to the priests.' And as they went, they were cleansed" (Luke 17:14). *And as they went.* How powerful.

Each day we must thank God for answers that are under way even though there are no outward, visible signs. We must live by faith and be thankful.

But only one of the ten returned to thank Jesus for his healing. In verses 15–19 we read: "One of them, when he saw he was healed, came back, praising God in a loud voice. He threw himself at Jesus' feet and thanked him—and he was a Samaritan. Jesus asked, 'Were not all ten cleansed? Where are the other nine? Has no one returned to give praise to God except this foreigner?' Then he said to him, 'Rise and go; your faith has made you well.'"

Here is that *believe* thing again. Give thanks to God for answers—even though there are no outward, visible signs. We needed to integrate our faith with an unceasing, resounding thankfulness, 24/7. Lord help us always to remember these three lessons:

- God knows what you need even before you ask (Matthew 6:8).
- God expects us to act out our faith. Their faith made them well. They proved this by heading to the priests while they still had leprosy. The passage says, "as they went, they were cleansed" (Luke 17:14).
- We must be grateful when He answers our prayers. If not, we could lose this blessing. How difficult would that be? All because we did not express proper gratitude.

"Expressing gratitude to human benefactors is common courtesy, and God expects no less," says Ed Strauss.[3]

Voskamp's words permeate my heart, "Jesus counts thanksgiving as integral in a faith that saves. We only enter into the full life if our faith gives thanks. Thanksgiving is inherent to a true salvation experience; thanksgiving is necessary to live the well, whole, fullest life."[4]

"Let the peace of Christ rule in your hearts, since as members of one body you were called to peace. And be thankful" (Colossians 3:15). Now that you have learned this, be peaceful to one another.

CHAPTER 33
PRESENCE IN ACTION

*One can never pay in gratitude; one can only
pay "in kind" somewhere else in life.*
—Anne Morrow Lindbergh

*Feeling gratitude isn't born in us—it's something we
are taught, and in turn we teach our children.*
—Joyce Brothers

They came with their trucks, vans, and SUVs and descended on our
narrow street. There were rakes, shovels, pitchforks, and fat toolboxes.
The driveway was already full of the four yards of bark that was delivered
the day before.

"Where should we park?" was a natural question. We have such a
close-knit neighborhood—a virtual family you might say—so, "go on
over to Rob's driveway," or "Elsie won't mind."

Once the vehicles were parked and the equipment in hand, the
teaming group of three families locked on the bark. This wheelbarrow
went one way, that wheelbarrow went another. Each was full to the
brim with thick, moist clumps of bark that would freshen up the sections
of landscaping.

This home in the "Key West without the chickens" neighborhood
sat on the corner of a tiny lot among a row of cottages built sometime

around World War I. There have been numerous remodels done by other owners over those years, with the last one that included a new roof and exterior siding. The house itself is old, but from the outside, it looks new. The fresh layer of bark will complete the picture.

Monica Gravenhof had been planning this gift to us for weeks. They were coordinating which weekend would work best for all three families and their children.

Chris did not join the barking party. I know he wanted to be there. Over the years, the two of us have gotten very adept at hauling and spreading. I'd haul; he'd spread. There were many sarcastic jokes over those years that he got the better end of the project. But spreading is not a job for a 2 in Follow Thru. I lose energy very fast for that job. If you want my sustainable energy, then it will need to be something that requires physical effort and moving. Years before we'd owned a home that required ten yards of bark—all needing to be hauled, dumped and spread by the end of the day.

It was calming to be within this circle of laughter, orders, and obedience. "Work on this section," or "they could use your help around front." I stopped my activity at one point to see him looking out the window of the back door. His blank eyes told the entire story. A week ago, he'd heard there was likely a recurrence of the tumor. There would be much more testing that he'd go through during the coming weeks. He couldn't get comfortable. We'd scheduled time with the palliative care team to go forward with medication for energy, sleep, and pain. Today he had throbbing headaches. As I locked onto his face, I imagined him thinking, *My yard will look great for my wake.*

How do we express our gratitude for this? Your time, your care, your concern. Showing up in ways that say, "I get you." Monica knows that Chris has a need for this pristine, finished look. She knows if he were well, he'd be out there on his knees, carefully smoothing each clump to cover the area in just the right way. This was a "church rally" of the greatest kind. We can never, ever, express the feeling of gratitude we had for these three families on that day—the Gravenhofs, the Rutherfords, and the Van Gelders. But we certainly can say it: "We thank you all from the bottom of our hearts."

I am the Lord, the God of all mankind. Is anything too hard for me?

Jeremiah 32:27

PART 7
EXPECT A MIRACLE

CHAPTER 34

DO YOU BELIEVE IN MIRACLES?

Miracles seem to attest to the presence of a loving and compassionate God, one who wants to help us, who wants to speak to us and encourage us.
—Eric Metaxes

Faith doesn't make sense, it makes miracles.
—Tony Evans

Those infamous words. Spoken by Al Michaels in Lake Placid, New York. It was February 22, 1980, at the Olympic Center, site of the men's hockey medal-round game that evening. Eighty-five hundred people were there to watch and hear the words we will never forget. The clock is counting down, eight seconds, five seconds. During training, Herb Brooks, the coach, would ask them, "Who do you play for?"

"USA."

Can you believe it? In the match versus Russia, USA is ahead. The winners will have the chance to advance and contend for the gold medal. Now it's three seconds. Pandemonium erupts. Team USA will hold the lead. One second. "Do you believe in miracles?"[1]

There is a home in Lake Geneva, Wisconsin, called the "Expect a Miracle" home. My sister-in-law, Donna, grew up in Williams Bay,

Wisconsin, on the western shore of Lake Geneva and focused my attention to this one theme: expect a miracle.

Visitors have access to a pathway all around Lake Geneva. An Indian treaty signed in 1833 guarantees public access to the path in perpetuity. What foresight was that! I am sure some of the homeowners do not like the in perpetuity clause, but the "Expect a Miracle" home has created a welcoming atmosphere by painting inspirational quotes all along the rails surrounding the path on this property. One of those quotes is, "peace to all who enter here." When you enter the space, you are encouraged to wish for a miracle. They have placed a bell along the path for people to stop and ring it and wish for something better in their lives. I have never been along the path in this area but have seen the home from the street. People say it is a beautiful place that provides you with hope—a way to connect and to meditate.

Jesus's first miracle was at the wedding at Cana. "When the wine was gone, Jesus' mother said to him, 'They have no more wine.' 'Dear woman, why do you involve me?' Jesus replied, 'My time has not yet come.' His mother said to the servants, 'Do whatever he tells you'" (John 2:3–5). Isn't this just perfect. She expected the miracle. She knew. She believed. She couldn't wait to see what would happen. Can't you just picture this scene. Jesus tells her, "my time has not yet come," and without missing a beat, she turns to the servants and says, "Do whatever he tells you."

"I submit to you that one of the reasons we don't see more miracles is because we don't expect more miracles," writes Dutch Sheets.[2]

We need to ring the bell. We need to express the desire for something better in our lives. We must take the initiative. We must pray big. We might, in fact, need to call our mother! We must believe, like Mary.

> Jesus said to the servants, "Fill the jars with water"; so they filled them to the brim. Then he told them, "Now draw some out and take it to the master of the banquet." They did so, and the master of the banquet tasted the water that had been turned into wine. He did not realize where it had come from, though the servants who had drawn the water knew. Then he called the bridegroom

aside and said, "Everyone brings out the choice wine first and then the cheaper wine after the guests have had too much to drink; but you have saved the best till now." This, the first of his miraculous signs, Jesus performed at Cana in Galilee. He thus revealed his glory, and his disciples put their faith in him (John 2:7–11).

Thomas Moore, in *Writing in the Sand*, says:

> The sheer humanity in this story is part of its message: Jesus responds to his mother's concern and offers a first glance at his teaching during a party, over something as ordinary as wine running out. At the same time, the wedding party represents the current human condition—our vitality, complexity, and spirit—is running out. The change of water to wine signifies a much deeper kind of change in the human spirit— from plain consciousness to an intoxicating vision. It is the central theme of the Gospels: go through a change of vision and discover life in all its abundance and intensity.[3]

> Expect to see miracles—and you will. Miracles are not always visible to the naked eye, but those who *live by faith* can see them clearly.[4]

A miracle is really a violation of the rules of experience. Vessels of water filled to the brim do not instantly turn into Far Niente. But a miracle defies all logic. While Chris and I continued to have setbacks and complications, transformation was beginning to be real and visible.

After a scheduled PET scan on May 6, we decided to venture to downtown Holland to see all the tulips in bloom on Eighth Street. We stopped along the way for Chris to rest and captured a beautiful picture with hundreds of pink tulips in their prime right behind him. Then, we made our way down the street to one of our favorite spots—The Seasoned Home. This is a shop where you can buy fresh spices by the ounce. There are also sure to be sampling tables for seasoned dips and specialty products. He landed on the pretzels and couldn't stop eating them. It was the first food I'd seen him eat by mouth in months. At first, both of us were overwhelmed at his appetite and desire to eat. It seemed unquestionably a miracle. But as time went on, I sensed this was just not right. Once we were home, his blood test confirmed that his sugar levels again were spiking out of control. He had had to suspend taking his diabetes medicine for twenty-four hours prior to the procedure. We needed to turn this around. After consulting with his PCP, back to the emergency room we went to get what we hoped would be a shot of insulin, to again get his diabetes under control.

The next few weeks were a roller coaster. The neck swelling on the left side of his throat continued to be a concern. The PET scan results showed that the tumor was not totally gone, and that the likely next step would now need to be surgery, since he couldn't go into a second round of chemo and radiation so soon after the first round. Chris was devastated. We were scheduled to meet with Dr. Prince in Ann Arbor to get the official next step: "Let's do another biopsy just to be sure." The biopsy was scheduled for May 28. The month of May seemed to be a different doctor visit each day. Dr. Hulst, Dr. Gribben, Dr. Prince, and now to see Dr. Edlund. It was always so encouraging to me to be able to tag along on these visits because he was the vocally optimistic one on the team. He served as a true encourager when Chris's mood and outlook could have turned completely negative. We were able to view the PET scan results and see that the tumor was significantly reduced, but there were still questions. We headed into a time of fasting and prayer for insight.

It was time for another diversion. Our two sons in Chicago have birthdays three days apart—May 27 and May 30. What better diversion than a birthday party. So, we planned a trip to Chicago for the day. Chris was beginning to eat and drink a few things, so both of us were looking forward to going to Chinatown, and a real meal out. But it was not to happen. Once we got there, Chris became very weak and had no energy to manage one more step. He stayed on the couch and slept; the rest of us went out to celebrate and sample some new flavors and selections but mostly just to laugh and be together.

CHAPTER 35
TIME LINE OF A MIRACLE

The singular importance of willpower in determining one's fate in life cannot be overstated.
—*Dr. Timothy Paterick*

My greatest point is my persistence. I never give up in a match. However down I am, I fight until the last ball. My list of matches shows that I have turned a great many so-called irretrievable defeats into victories.
—*Bjorn Borg*

These are the text messages to my sister-in-law, Donna Mantey.

1/21: "Needs to stay eating regular food. Dr. chastised him."

1/24: "Faith (ahhh). Blizzard. Need to stop and rest in the presence of Jesus."

1/25: "Tumor is shrinking. Cold day. Quiet day, inside. Angels, angels everywhere."

1/26: "To church today with difficulty. Kiss my mother for me on her birthday. I sure could use some family close by right now."

1/28: "You, Donna, my CEO—Chief Encouragement Officer. 4th Chemo."

1/29: "Work. Sweet work abounds. Thank you, Jesus."

2/3: "*Jesus Calling* right on."

2/4: "Jud's 93rd Birthday. Took picture at oncology place. Dr. says Chris is doing great!"

2/7: "Ara for the weekend. Drive to Michigan City."

2/9: "Back to train."

2/11: "Very emotional day. Radiation oncologist 'could not feel the tumor or see it visually anymore. It is basically gone. Now we just need to do cleanup.'"

2/13: "Stayed in Fremont."

2/14: "Peace. What a beautiful feeling. Happy Valentine's Day. So many prayers answered. I am thanking the Lord for answers to prayers that are already in the works but just not evident yet. How sweet that feels."

2/18: "Things going downhill very fast. So weary. No energy at all. Sick all the time. I'm painting the living room. Took a team to get him to radiation. So many drugs. Getting Ritalin. 7th Chemo. Tolerating it so well we might as well do 8, Dr. said. He has zero energy. Got blood work and everything looks great."

2/20: "Will need a miracle for Chris to make it to next Thursday. He is miserable. Only 5 more radiations and one chemo on Tuesday left."

2/21: "Only 4 more treatments. We are counting down triumphantly. The Lord will heal. We are confident."

2/21: "Not getting enough hydration. Working on it."

2/22: "Dramatic changes. In Emergency Room. Pray."

2/22: "Blood sugar issues. 386 at 6 a.m. this morning. How can this be when things are so monitored?"

2/22: "Cat scan to rule out serious issues. Trying to rule out clots. Thinks he's going to die. PTL—everything is fine. No clot. No stroke. He has to walk steady before they will release him. He is borderline being admitted."

2/22: "Geoff and Ellen came. Had dinner at Irish Pub in Saugatuck."

2/22: "Not tolerating anything by mouth. Don't know what to do. Good visit with E & G."

2/23: "Back in ER. Pray without ceasing. In chapel. Genesis 35:9. New name. Tribute to stay close to God despite life's disappointments. On the mend. Drug reaction to about 10 different medications he is on."

2/24: "Hemoglobin low. Need to stay another day. Transfusion soon."

2/25: "Going home from hospital. New way to feed that will be better for Chris. No more chemo. Done. Home, ahhhh."

2/26: "Tough winter conditions."

2/28: "Dr. Edlund encouraged in spite of recent setbacks. Dr. Hulst to keep diabetes in check."

2/28: "Photo shoot for new website! Need more fun!"

2/28: "Need break from blowing snow."

3/2: "What a joy to worship our Lord and King! Motivated to stay hydrated. He watered plants and cleaned up dead leaves. Not shaking a rug, but better. Color in face. Just 2 more days of treatment. We rest in God's almighty plan."

3/3: "Roof leak. Ugh. Took Chris for treatment."

3/4: "Final treatment! Crossed the finish line. Now for healing and recoup and reenergize."

3/5: "I'm feeling particularly full of God's abundant love."

3/7: "Decatur, IL. Client there. 50 degrees weather, ahhhh. Ara for weekend."

3/9: "Great sermon on Grace. Chris down 6 pounds???? Everything so volatile."

3/10: "Trying to drink water. Can taste chocolate. Great progress."

3/11: "Late meeting with Chemo Dr. Very weak. See what he has to say."

3/12: "We need prayers."

3/13: "4 degrees outside. Dr. says Chris will be at his worst, but things should turn around."

3/14: "To coffee today at JPs with friends. To the plant shop for a little spring picture with Jim Jonker."

3/15: "Back to the plant shop."

3/16: "Frigidly cold."

3/21: "Feeling discouraged. Yesterday so weak. Need prayers. Need to keep getting calories. Blood sugar under control. Isaiah 40:28–31."

3/27: "Massive coughing spell. Back in ER."

3/27: "Loosened up neck and throat tissue. Big setback. Feels he won't make it. Prayers to stay positive and strong."

3/27: "Stable, but being transferred to GR, St. Mary's. Blood transfusion. Very low hemoglobin. Kidney questions. Habakkuk 3:17–19. Zephaniah 3:17."

3/28: "Setback could have been the set up for his comeback. Renewed energy. What a friend we have in Jesus."

4/2: "Losing heart. See radiologist. We like him and respect what he says."

4/2: "*Jesus Calling* trilogy on peace, peace, peace. Ara visit gave Chris a boost. Dr. asking him to challenge himself more. No appetite."

4/5: "Lost whole breakfast. Prayer warrior prayed over Chris."

4/6: "Ran 7 miles. Church. Both help me maintain a clear mind, peace and continual reliance and trust in God's will. Isaiah 26: 3 from *The Message*: completely whole, steady on their feet, keep at it, don't quit. Whole chapter of Isaiah 26. Colossians 3. Grace. New postures of the heart and new practices of the mouth."

4/8: "Tackled outstanding medical bills. Sorted things out that are overwhelming. Baby is kicking regularly. Masters Tournament this weekend. Bills of $900, and $760, and $382, and $570, and on and on. Insurance coordinating. Answer to prayer."

4/12: "Masters Tournament. Jordan Spieth."

4/16: "Calling in palliative care. Exodus 14. Praying for the right answers. Need to get him comfortable."

4/18: "Dr. Strabbing: likely recurrence of the tumor. Need a miracle for dead tumor to vanish. Potential for surgery. Not feeling up to it. Will be doing lots more testing in the next few weeks. So uncomfortable."

4/19: "James 1:12. Watching golf and remembering Harbour Town Hilton Head."

4/21: "Slept through the night. Coughing less and less. Thinks today he can beat this thing."

4/22: "SNAFU—Rx ready for pickup in NEW HOLLAND, PA!! Dr. Gribben says healing takes time. Do not dismay. Could have been a false alarm. He's seen this before. This is his job. New medication for energy, sleep, and pain."

4/24: "We will see what God has planned for today."

4/25: "Thank you for your unwavering devotion to us."

4/26: "Too many headaches. Small group from another church to administer to us. Monica's small group. Organized raking, cleaning, barking our yard. It looks marvelous. Fixed our broken fountain."

4/27: "Spark of life today."

5/2: "Cancer is stressful. Root canal for me. If not one thing, now another."

5/4: "Back in ER. Very, very, weak. Praying circles around Chris. Waiting for CAT scan. Being transferred to St. Mary's hospital. God will keep in perfect peace those whose minds are stayed on Him!"

5/5: "St. Mary's. No Dr. No ENT. Just holding it all together. Dr. Gribben later tonight. Staying overnight. Neck swelling other side."

5/6: "Pray for calm. He needs calm. Wonderful day. Fervent prayers avail much. You my dear sister have poured your heart out and we are so grateful. What a miracle. So much transformation over the last three days. We live as Third Day Christians."

5/8: "On a roll. What a miracle! Working on real eating. Chicken soup. Mostly broth, but real food nonetheless."

5/11: "Chris to church in first time since ?? February?"

5/13: "Big week. Dr. Hulst; Dr. Prince; Dr. Edlund."

5/13: "Rough news. Tumor not totally gone. Next step likely is surgery. Chris is devastated."

5/14: "Drinking out of a coffee cup. Psalms 31:24."

5/15: "In Ann Arbor. Big day. Big prayers. But we know we have a mighty God. Biopsy for 5/28. First real quasi meal—tea, egg drop soup, cashew shrimp."

5/16: "Dr. Edlund optimistic, but cautious. Biopsy 5/28. PET scan. Tumor significantly reduced. Still questions though."

5/19: "Going into a time of fasting and prayer for insight."

5/24: "Trip to Chicago for A & G birthdays. Great lunch out with Mary Beth and Mary. Long day."

5/25: "Boat ride. Jim and Judy, Chris' friends from high school, stopped by."

6/8: "Chris started reading a book."

6/12: "The Lord's name is a Strong Tower. The righteous run to Him and are safe. Proverbs 18:10."

6/13: "Nothing happening with baby. Getting head in right position."

6/16: "Calm with Ellen and baby. Nothing."

6/17: "Throat swollen."

6/18: "Second biopsy post treatment. Zach took him. Ecclesiastes Chapter 3. Today he feels his mother watching over him. She died on June 18th. She always said, "nothing bad lasts forever." Accelerated analysis. No cancer. Just radiation irritation. So many precautions."

6/18: "New Rx to help swelling and irritation."

6/20: "Ultrasound. No signs she's coming today. 7 lbs., 3 oz. if born today. Please hurry baby girl Crittenden."

6/22: "Dr. Lou Lotz—Covenant Rainbow—Revelations 4. The rainbow is for joy. God's memory of his promise in Genesis. It is a visible sign of his invisible grace. In Revelations the visual is that God is clothed in this covenant promise—the rainbow. No Baby Girl Crittenden. Nothing happening."

6/27: "Chris is gaining confidence that he is getting better."

6/28: "Ellen @ the hospital. Breaking water soon."

6/29: "4:40 a.m. Central time. Caroline Isabel Crittenden. What a boost to the healing process."

7/11: "Landmark day! To the driving range to hit a bucket of balls. Small bag, each! A big step."

7/18: "Want to cry. Chris asked if I wanted to go out for dinner. Such a long time since we've been to a restaurant."

7/21: "This is the day. Here we are. Expect a Miracle home in Lake Geneva."

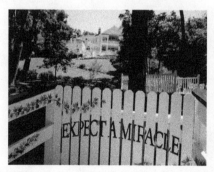 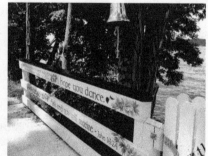

Expect a Miracle Home

If you have never listened to Jim Valvano's ESPY Award speech, you are missing out on one of the all-time ever, greatest motivational speeches on the planet. Jim Valvano, legendary basketball coach, has touched our lives through the V Foundation—dedicated to saving lives by helping to find a cure for cancer. The foundation is an advocate for cancer research and to create an urgent awareness among all Americans of the importance of the war on cancer.

Jimmy V lost his fight to cancer but encourages us through these words:

> We should do three things every day of our life. Number one is laugh. You should laugh every day. Number two is think. We should spend some time in thought. And, number three is you should have your emotions moved to tears ... Cancer can take away all of my physical abilities. It cannot touch my mind, it cannot touch my heart, and it cannot touch my soul ... Don't give up. Don't ever give up.[1]

The power to harness your will makes all the difference between life and death.
Pause and review the time line of our miracle. It wasn't an instantaneous, *take up your bed and walk.* It wasn't immediate water into wine after hearing *do what he says.* It took months. It was the cha-cha, as some would like to say. Euphoria one day, disaster the next—weeks on end. Don't give up. Don't ever give up.

CHAPTER 36
THE MIRACLE OF NEW LIFE

To witness the birth of a child is our best opportunity to experience the meaning of the word miracle.
—*Paul Carvel*

I don't know who my grandfather was. I am more concerned to know what his grandson will be.
—*Abraham Lincoln*

Expect: regard (something) as likely to happen; believe that (someone or something will arrive soon.

Synonyms: anticipate, await, look for, hope for, look forward to, contemplate.[1]

Our story includes one of the most fabulous events that can occur in all of humankind. Truly a miracle. The birth of a child.

June 29: This was an incredible day. Well, June 28 was hectic with Ellen going into labor on that Saturday morning. Geoff and I kept texting away throughout the day and into the night, and then our beautiful granddaughter, Caroline Isabel Crittenden, was born in the early hours of June 29, 2014. What a memorable day, as this is the birth date of my grandmother, Anna. And now to have a granddaughter born on the exact day of my grandmother's birthday—the circle of life in all its glory.

The confirmation that she had arrived triggered urgent action. We must get to Chicago immediately so that he can hold her, look her in the eyes, and touch this miracle of new life. Just like the woman who reached out to touch Jesus's robe, the mere intention of the touch became the means of her healing. I needed to be the conduit to get him within proximity to make the touch. With a good understanding of the location of the hospital, I was able to find a hotel just a block away. Even that small walk proved to be almost insurmountable. We would walk a few steps; then he would need to stop. Once we got into the spacious lobby of the hospital, even then, he would have to stop and sit down to muster the energy to make it to the bank of elevators.

As we rode up the elevator, I could see the anticipation on his face. He had so many doubts that he would be alive to see her, but he had made it to this day—her day of birth. He would now see her face-to-face.

Caroline, "we'll call her CeCe," put a spark in Chris's heart and in his outlook. Those first few hours with them on that Sunday morning are nestled in our hearts forever.

May you live to see your children's children. Peace be upon Israel. (Psalm 128:6)

Could this possibly be the turning point we needed? Yes, I believe.

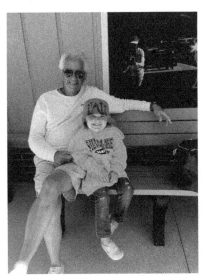

Grandpa and CeCe

CHAPTER 37
THE MIRACLE OF A HEALING PRACTICE

No pain, no palm; no thorns, no throne; no gall, no glory; no cross, no crown.
—William Penn

Put your ear down close to your soul and listen hard.
—Anne Sexton

Have you ever overheard someone sharing something with another person? What if that something you overheard could be life changing for someone else. This was the case for Jessica Barendse. Jessica is the daughter of our longtime friends Mike and Julie. She was working at a chiropractor's office in Hudsonville when she overheard one of their patients share with a nurse about the medical research she was involved in during the fall of 2015. It went something like this: "We do acupuncture for throat cancer patients posttreatment to help them regain the function to develop saliva." Jessica's ears perked up with the words "throat cancer" and "posttreatment." After this patient's treatment session, she was determined to walk her back up to the front lobby. She was hoping it would give her a chance to ask more questions and get more details. What she learned in those few minutes of interaction was that a current phase of the study was just wrapping up, and they were ready to work with another cohort. Based on what she heard, she didn't quite know if this was a good fit with Chris's current state, but what could it hurt to share this opportunity with him? Jessica was currently attending Grand Valley State University and taking a class on various aspects of research and what makes a good case study. Because of this class and what she was learning, her radar was up on this type of research. The patient gave Jessica the phone number for Chris to call to determine his fit with this study and if he might benefit in his posttreatment phase as part of those chosen for the upcoming cohort.

Jessica couldn't contain herself and called Chris right away. "I don't know if it will pan out to be anything, but it's worth you checking it out." This is from one Fact Finder to another. Chris called the number and was invited to come to a meeting to share his history, vitals, treatments, and current phase of recovery. He was accepted.

We look back on this tip and see it not as an overheard conversation but definitely the will of God to place Jessica in that very spot. Finding this opportunity for Chris to be involved was truly a miracle. It was the right place, right time, and most certainly God-driven.

One of the circumstances of radiation in the throat and neck area is that the salivary glands are affected by the radiation. Patients going through radiation treatments may never regain or are slow to regain the ability to create saliva. This was an acupuncture study to bring back the function of saliva development.

The most common forms of combating dry mouth are sucking lozenges or chewing gum. There are several disadvantages in that they must be used constantly, and that the effects are often short-lived.[1] Chris was going to be a part of a case study in Grand Rapids to determine the benefits of acupuncture to improve saliva production. He was going to be a part of a spit test!

He went to a medical research facility once a week for about eight weeks, he recalls. He had to spit for them three times. One at the outset, one in the middle, and one at the end to determine if this treatment generated an increase in his flow of saliva.

I remember specifically where the technician inserted each needle. He put thirteen needles into various parts of my body—head, hands, and legs. They were inside each ear, on each side of my ankles, legs and wrists. The odd one went into my chin. I needed to be very still so they wouldn't fall out.

The technician wasn't unkind or abrupt but was succinctly clear that he couldn't comment on anything. "I can't have any communication with you," he said. Chris was not told during the acupuncture treatments if he was part of the group that received the "active" treatment, or if he was in the placebo group. He just felt good about being involved.

Whether it was the treatment, or the idea of the treatment, Chris began to produce more saliva. This in turn created a greater appetite, which created the desire to eat, which put the whole digestive process back in the saddle, so to speak.

We were not privy to all the details of this program and the rigors of this clinical trial during the treatments, but Chris's water was truly turned into wine by thirteen needles, inserted weekly, in an environment of low light and soft, relaxing music, prone in a big, cushy recliner. *Listen to the unheard and see the invisible.*

CHAPTER 38
THE MIRACLE OF LOVE

You come to love not by finding the perfect person,
but by seeing an imperfect person perfectly.
—Sam Keen

It is love, not reason, that is stronger than death.
—Thomas Mann

She spent the rest of the afternoon with him. First she asked for a basin, got some hot water, and shaved him. Then she found a nurse to help her dress him. In his own clothes, clean-shaven, his hair combed, he seemed suddenly almost whole again, a *person* instead of a patient. Delia thought she could actually feel a difference in the way the nurses and aides treated him when they came into the room. She helped to feed him too. Spooning the mush he was allowed into his mouth.

Mostly, though, she just sat by him, sometimes saying a few words, more often humming or singing. The time seemed to pass with a glacial slowness. When Tom dozed and she could relax—she could walk in the hallway for a bit or go into the bathroom and splash water on her face—Delia felt a gratitude so profound it was almost physical.[1]

Some people describe love as something powerful, spiritual, and even primal—a kind of love that might be likened to a "glimpse of heaven."[2] Others describe it as intense, impulsive, intimate. There are a multitude of great words that describe love: devotion, desire, companion, caring, tenderness, fondness, nearness, happiness, friendship, affection, adoration, romance, infatuation.

My love for Chris is all-consuming. I want to be near him and with him. Talking and laughing—so often laughing. He has a very quick wit and sees his goal in life is to make me smile and laugh. Laughter is 90 percent of our love. We are great companions because we like the same things: golf, football, biking, decorating. If I'm shopping, he will be looking for outfits I might try on. He has great taste. If the house needs a new pillow or decoration, we spot just what it needs at the same time. We do this together.

Love is someone who wakes you up in the middle of the night to do the play-by-play and the full-blown commentary on a Green Bay Packers football game that you wanted desperately to watch but were too tired to stay up and watch, and you aren't the least bit angry that you are now wide awake, and there is zero chance you can go back to sleep. That is a comfortable love.

We love our children unconditionally because we practice the actions of love with them throughout their lives. But we fail to practice the actions of love with our spouse throughout our marriage. Feelings do follow actions. As I tore open the bandages, and as I pumped the fluids through his life tube, my love grew deeper and broader and wider. I echo Timothy Keller's words: "But the passion we share now differs from the thrill we had then like a noisy but shallow brook differs from a quieter but much deeper river."[3]

Love is wonderful yet scary, passionate yet loyal, complicated yet simple, tender yet playful, silent yet loud, difficult yet easy, indescribable yet intuitive, compulsive yet compassionate, hurt yet healed, romantic yet realistic, together yet not forfeiting selfhood, submitting yet not giving in, eternal yet filled with today—the here and the now, this very moment. Love is giving your whole heart away—every piece, every cell, every iota—knowing that it will be broken, aching, and smashed to smithereens. Love is being so connected that you get your beloved, and he gets you. Love is an enigma, a beautiful mystery. Love is extending yourself and refreshing the other. Love is knowing and doing something about it.

We have been blessed with the miracle of love.

*I wait for the Lord, my soul waits,
and in his word I put my hope.*

Psalm 130:5

PART 8

WE WAIT

CHAPTER 39
CHICAGO MARATHON 2017

God's definition of success is really one of significance, the
significant difference our lives can make in the lives of others.
—*Tony Dungy*

No one is useless in the world who
lightens the burden of another.
—*Charles Dickens*

It seemed like a pretty good idea at the time. But that was back in November when the notice appeared in my email. You've been selected for a "lottery entry" into the Bank of America Chicago Marathon. What does that mean? Well, if I jump on this today and enter, pay my $195, I might get selected to participate. What can it hurt? So, I did. The original intent was to recommit to my running schedule. My right hip had developed serious pain, and I wasn't running consistently. My training was off and on, altogether very sporadic. The sixteen-week training schedule might just be the incentive I needed.

In December I got the notification that I was "in" again. I would be running in my eighth marathon at age sixty-three. Could I even hope to have a goal of under four hours and thirty minutes?

The severe pain in my right hip continued. I was really running and training injured, and I needed some expert advice. In July I decided if I was committed to running this, then I would need the help and support of a physical therapist. The words to me that I remember were, "I see. You can run, but you can't walk. I can help you." After we had worked together for several weeks his words went like this: "I'll clear you to run it, I'm just not that excited about it for you."

What does running injured feel like? First, you just don't want to get out of bed in the morning and make the effort. In the words of my physical therapist, "I'm just not that excited about it." That bothers me because running has been such a meaningful part of my life. Once I get going, I don't feel specific pain, but it also isn't a feeling of running free and light. There's a sense that I am carrying a weight that I want to put down. The weight is real because the pain is real, but the weight is also the self-talk that is going on in my head. What if I land wrong? Do I have the strength to stay in balance? If I lose my balance, do I have the strength to manage the fall? I have fallen a few times. One time was especially bad, with the underside of my chin serving as the brake pad. Because of those instances, I am always thinking, *Will I fall and break a bone this time?* It's just one faulty step, and "down goes Frazier."[1] So, it is a feeling of hesitancy. That is how I might describe it.

And now, I am here, in Chicago, in October, fully committed to this challenge. But not at all confident. Not at all excited. I am hesitant. The temperatures are expected to climb close to eighty degrees, with no cloud cover. It will be sunny. Two of the worst things a runner can hear—hot and full sun. There was a third kink in the equation now too. The runners would have staggered start times. I would go out in wave 3 of the starters. My start time now would be 8:35 CDT. That's sixty-five minutes behind the normal start. Wow. Nine thirty-five in my head. I am seldom ever running at 9:35 a.m. That would certainly be on the tail end of a very long training run. I would have my sites locked on home at that point. Where will the sun be by then? Oh, but all those things we will deal with on Sunday morning.

Walking to the race on Sunday is always fun. There is so much activity, and it's always nice to connect with one or two runners. This year it was a man from England. We chatted about our running history. I ran this marathon. He ran that one. "Are you ready," he asked. I nodded and said, "Yeah." We talked about the weather. It was nothing in particular that was memorable but someone to walk with and talk with and keep the edge off. Once at the area to load into the corral, I realized it would be a long wait. Several people were sitting on the curb, and I decided to do the same to take some pressure off my legs. I talked with a man who had some of the same concerns—body aches, hot temps, and sunny. I thought about moving away so the conversation could switch to a more positive topic, but I decided to stay and keep the banter going.

At that moment I came to realize my focus. I would run the "race of cancer." While I was running, I would put myself totally in the mindset of someone with this disease, needing to endure the pain, go through the struggle, and stay committed to fight. Comparing my hip injury and cancer are not even remotely close, but it was the best comparison I could make at that moment.

This made the wait so much easier. I immediately began to recall the time of waiting we had with Chris. From October with the diagnosis to January when treatments started seemed like a lifetime. The ticking time bomb analogy popped to mind. How did he deal with this? What did he do to keep sane? How did he handle the wait? Did I totally miss the time of desperation he was in? Was I a good wife? Did I brush him off? Was I there holding his hand? What was it like for him when he got fitted with the mask he would use during radiation? Chris Mortensen, another throat cancer survivor, referred it to the mask that Hannibal Lector was seen wearing in *Silence of the Lambs*.[2] All these questions and more starting streaming into my mind. I was surrounded by a sea of people, but I felt so very alone.

The gun went off and the elite group in the first wave was out of the blocks. I heard the name Galen Rupp[3] and silently hoped he would do well. I liked him and knew he'd had some disappointments over the years. I had already managed to navigate the toilets, so the only thing remaining to do was determine when I would start drinking the last of the water I had brought along. Why did we have so many hydration issues? Did we not know? Were we stupid? Why wasn't I as focused as I am today on when and how much liquid Chris was getting through his tube?

Countdown. It's finally happening. The long wait and now the gun.

We are off. I am in the corral with a group of runners that have close to the same ability. What do you got today, Mari? My last finish, in 2014, was 4:24:21. Can I perform well today? Will I be able to run through the pain? What will I have to do to make it across the finish line? That is the most important thing.

At the start of the race everyone is fresh and excited for the journey. Hope abounds. We've come with extra layers, and now most of those are strewn throughout the road. My mind drifts to memories of great times running, especially in Chicago. We are heading up Columbus Avenue, and I immediately think of Marathon #1, in 2006, running with my son. We stayed together at the Fairmont Chicago Millennium Park the night before. I can see the Fairmont up ahead now. What excitement we both had to do well. I focus back on the present and see the enormous crowds of cheering fans on both sides of the street. How great it is to have family and friends along in your journey. Many are there at the beginning. Be thankful and ask them to stay to the finish. So many want to be with you at the start, but make sure you position them well along the way. I know I will see my family at Mile 6, Mile 9, Mile 17, Mile 22, Mile 25, and maybe one or two other times. But for sure, I know they will be there. And I will be anticipating their waves, their smiles, and listen for "Go, Mom." It will be beautiful. I want to make it for them.

The early miles the temperatures are still cool and the sun not yet high in the sky. The tall buildings block most of the sun, and the pace is great and the effort minimal. *This is going to be easy. I'll make it, I'm sure.* At that moment I heard a most special whisper, *I will put My thoughts in your mind and My song in your heart. Run it and tell it—the crowds, the signs, and the journey.*

The signs of the fans stuck out to me the most in the first two miles. How our words matter so much to those needing encouragement. **BRENDA—Don't Cave.** How meaningful. It is important to get your loved one through the treatment phase. Chris only had one shot at it. There is no round two for chemo and radiation. Make it count. If you aren't doing it right, there is no alternative.

Chris in his first weeks of treatment was methodical. He was always on time. Never late. He was diligent to do everything exactly as ordered. Literally. He did not cave. He excelled.

I recalled Chris's period when he began to have difficulties making it through the day. He didn't want to feed himself. He was sleeping twenty hours a day. He seemed listless. He needed to be hospitalized and couldn't finish the last chemo treatment. As caregivers, we need to stay alert to all signs so our loved ones won't cave in.

The bridge I'm on is covered with red carpet. It feels soft when my foot lands. In treatment we are made to feel very special. Especially if you need to go to the Lemmon Holton Cancer Center for a PET scan. There is valet parking. The rooms are comfortable and airy. The patient's chair has every feature to control hot and cold, up and down, and any position in between. Or if you are admitted to the Lacks Cancer Center at Saint Mary's Hospital. I call it the Lacks Ritz. Both of these patientcentric facilities give you a five-star experience. As caregivers, how can we do this at home? I think about a red-carpet type experience I could have provided to Chris at home. Not just for a short spurt across the bridge, but for the whole twenty-six-mile journey. Was I sensitive to his needs for the right temperature, or was I always dialing down the thermostat? About now I am already feeling too warm, and it doesn't give me confidence for the remaining twenty-five miles. *My hip hurts. This will be a test.*

I make the turn onto State Street. I am familiar with these streets of Chicago. Since 1998 we have been coming to town regularly to visit our son, Ara. We most often get a different hotel and spend the weekend walking the Magnificent Mile, finding a new place to dine and just hanging out with each other. These are the streets that I have run, early on a Sunday morning during those weekends. Sometimes I head south through the Museum Campus and out to the lakeshore path. But most times I head north to Fullerton. I most enjoy the run up to Lincoln Park to see the Lincoln statue near the Chicago History Museum. The chiseled words of the second inaugural are there to remind us all:

> With malice toward none; with charity for all; with firmness in the right, as God gives us to see the right, let us strive on to finish the work we are in; to bind up the

nation's wounds; to care for him who shall have borne the battle, and for his widow, and his orphan; to do all which may achieve and cherish a just, and lasting peace, among ourselves, and with all nations.[4]

State Street. The marquee of the Chicago Theater. I know this. I know the shops and the landmarks. It feels good to be familiar. Keep focusing on the familiar. Familiarity removes anxiety. How did I help Chris navigate the unfamiliar? I was there with him when we went for the PET scans. I was there with him the first time we went to meet Dr. Prince at the University of Michigan Medical Center. Ann Arbor was familiar because Geoff was there for four years. We knew the streets we needed to be on and the lane we needed to be in to turn. Ann Arbor is crazy to get around in, but we knew it; we'd been there before.

And then I turned onto LaSalle and saw them. The banners. They were hanging from each of the lampposts. The faces of the greats. People like Greg Meyer, Joan Benoit-Samuelson, and Paula Radcliffe.[5] Over five hundred thousand athletes have finished this race since its inception in 1977. These were the faces of those we knew. Those who had gone first into uncharted waters on these streets in October. Those who have endured the heat and the sun like today, and even the cold, the rain, and the wind conditions of another time and another year. These banners gave me hope for my journey today. *You will make it. You will cross the finish line. You will survive. You are on LaSalle Street. Enjoy this moment.*

LaSalle Street has always been one of my favorite portions of the marathon run with the wide boulevard and crowds of people. It was on LaSalle Street in 2009 at mile four that I realized I had trained well and had some jump in my step, so I had better step it up. It was the turning point of that race. It is on LaSalle that I get invigorated by the music and the bands around the Moody Bible Institute. It is on LaSalle that I begin to sense a closeness to my family. I know where they will be. It is a tradition for Chris, Ara, and Geoff to be standing on the northwest corner of Fullerton. It is there that I will be kissed and sent on my way.

The weight of my decision came down hard when I crossed the half-marathon mark. *I have nothing left right now. Nothing. Just keep moving.*

Walk if you must. As I turned onto Adams Street, there was a small child offering licorice to the runners that would stop and take his gift. I was intrigued by his genuine care and concern for each of us. In his heart he believed that his gift, this piece of licorice, would have magical healing powers to boost our energy. I bent down to receive the gift. It brought back memories of a message from my mother: Receive the Gift and Enjoy the Gift. "When God puts you in a position that requires you to receive from another, do it with graciousness, with gratefulness, and with humility. Don't deny the other person the blessing of giving to you."[6]

"Hey, lady, lady, you need this. It will make you run faster. Lady, here you go. Eat my licorice. I want you to have it."

As I transition into Chinatown, I know it won't be long before Geoff and CeCe come into sight. I look up ahead, and there they are right on the corner of Wentworth. I'll need to swing to the outside lane to get over there. He's holding her, and I just want to connect, say hi, and linger for a few moments. We make eye contact, and I reach out to touch them, and I kiss CeCe on the cheek. Her immediate instinct is to brush her hand across her cheek displaying a need to "get that kiss off me." I'm hot, I'm sweaty, and possibly unrecognizable. Does she no longer know I'm her grandma? Does she want nothing to do with me because I have changed? Chris's looks changed a lot over the time that he was doing battle with this foe. Did I brush his kiss off my mouth when he had cancer breath? Was I kind and considerate to him when a putrid stench was pouring out of his mouth? Did I hold him close even though he was a totally different man than the one I fell in love with? *Mile marker 22, just four miles to go. I will make this if I must walk every step.* And that's about what I did to survive. Run, walk, run, walk.

I'm on the only stretch that runs on Michigan Avenue. My goal for my personal best 2009 run was "to be running down Michigan Avenue." On that day I was, but not today. This is another year and a different set of circumstances. And then I see a sign that says it all: **You Don't Know Me, But I Admire You.** Chris, I truly admire you for all you went through. Most of it silently, I might add. It was heavy-handed treatment you had to endure. Be an inspiration to others, and let them know they can make it too!

The finish is near, just up the cresting hill on Roosevelt, turn onto Columbus, and you will be done. You can go home. Or at least to the hotel. I do begin to sprint to the finish, mostly to stop the voices in my head reconciling how I will be able to make one more stretch, one more block, even one more step. I see the final sign on the course that puts a broad grin across my face: **YOU ARE GRITTY. THAT'S A LOT OF WORK FOR A FREE BANANA.**

And then it's over. No fanfare. No familiar faces shouting their hurrahs. Just over. Crossing the finish line wasn't euphoric or exhilarating. It wasn't emotional or even exciting. But it was satisfying, rewarding, and gratifying. The precise moment I stepped across the finish line was filled with joy. Pure, unadulterated joy. Everything the color of yellow exploded in my vision. *I have finished the race I set out to run.* In Paul's letter to Timothy: "I have fought the good fight, I have finished the race. I have kept the faith" (1 Timothy 4:7).

I reach out to accept the medal that each of us receives after we clear the finish line. Then the words from John Candy's character in *Cool Runnings*, one of the all-time feel-good movies ever—about the development of the Jamaican bobsled team—comes to mind: "A gold medal is a beautiful thing, but if you're not enough without it, you'll never be enough with it."[7] I can hang this around my neck today, and people throughout Chicago will stop and congratulate me, some may admire me, but they will not even begin to understand the full story. There were so many untold personal moments that I simply want to treasure deeply within my own heart while I am yet living. *It's just between you and Me.*

Now for the walk back to the hotel. Will my legs hold out to get me there? So, I just start walking north to find an opening out of the finishing chute, past the people handing out medals to other runners, past the aluminum foil blankets, past the tables and tables of bananas, bars, and bagels. I have run to remember, and I have run to sense in a very small way the emotional toll on the mind, the soul, and the body when you are sick on the inside, and now you must tackle the biggest fight of your life. I just kept walking. I just kept upright.

I passed the restricted area and found the first street out. A man was leaning up against the fence and shouted encouragement, "You didn't use it all up. Good for you that you have some left to get out of here. I can't move." *You must have the strength to get back down the mountain.* We were staying at the Allegro, and so I had several blocks to walk. My mindset was: *Choose the straightest path. Figure out now when to head north. Don't go farther than you need to.* About this time, I ran into a mother and a daughter, I presumed, both hunched over with a look of defeat as they just couldn't or wouldn't take one step more, for fear it was not the right direction. They had no idea where they were in relation to their hotel. I realized in a moment that neither had an ounce of energy to make the wrong move. I knew exactly what they were feeling. *Must have the strength to get back down the mountain.*

"Where are you staying," I asked.

"The Gray," came from each of them simultaneously.

My first thoughts were to say words of encouragement: "You are very close. Head this way till you get to Monroe, turn left on Monroe, and your hotel is on Monroe. You can't miss it. It's a few blocks, but you are very close. I need to go that way too. Would you like to walk together?" *Teamwork is critical.*

We must all help each other see that the end of the fight is very near, and you do have the energy to get there, even though you may not believe it in that moment. "Everyone helps his neighbor and says to his brother, 'Be strong!'" (Isaiah 41:6 ESV).

Chris and I found ourselves in an unbearable situation, and God's plan for us was for full and complete healing so that we could bear fruit.

CHAPTER 40
PRETTY WELL

Man's main task is to give birth to himself.
—Erich Fromm

What makes the desert beautiful is that somewhere it hides a well.
—Antoine de Saint-Exupéry

In the early 1990s we hosted a young woman from France as she did a summer internship at Haworth Corporation. It was announced at a Rotary meeting that this young woman needed a host family for four weeks that summer as a request from her Rotarian father in France. We had an extra bedroom, and it just seemed to be the right thing to do. Her name was Francoise. That summer we spent more time than we have ever before sitting around the dining room table over our evening meal, learning from her and she from us.

One evening, we went to a Hope Summer Repertory play: *Twelfth Night*. It was Ara, Francoise, and me. When the lights went up for admission, she leaned over to me and said, "I don't get it; it doesn't make any sense." Ara was just as quick with: "Don't feel bad; it's in English, and I don't get it either."

Francoise took it upon herself to be immersed in our language. She was captivated with words and jargon. This was a woman who could speak six languages fluently, so dialect came easily for her. Her big desire was to understand American slang. The word that perplexed her the most was *pretty*.

"What's with this word, *pretty*," she asked one day. "Things are pretty good, and things are pretty bad. I just don't get *pretty*." We were around the table for a pretty long time.

And so, I ask, "What's with this word *well*?" The dictionary shows there are a minimum of fifteen ways this word can be used:

1. In a good or satisfactory manner: our plans are going *well*.
2. Thoroughly, carefully, soundly: the problem is *well* understood.
3. In a moral or proper manner: to behave *well*.
4. Commendably, meritoriously, or excellently: a difficult task *well* handled.
5. With favor or approval: to think *well* of someone.
6. Comfortably or prosperously: to live *well*.
7. With great or intimate knowledge: to know a person *well*.
8. With good nature; without rancor: he took the joke *well*.
9. Come up as a liquid: tears *welled* up in her eyes.
10. In good health, sound in body and mind: I feel *well*.
11. Well-being; good fortune; success: to wish *well* to someone.
12. Wise or advantageous: it would be *well* to start early.
13. Used to express a range of emotions including surprise, anger, resignation, or relief: "*Well*, really, she had the audacity to say that!"
14. Natural source or abundant source: she is a *well* of information.
15. A deep place in the earth where water, oil, gas, or brine can be pulled up from: they dug a *well*.[1]

We don't need to be eloquent, effulgent, articulate, impeccable, flawless, loquacious. There are many words that evoke intense emotion with only four letters. As I finish this book, these are the words that I am now drawn to: able, aura, best, bond, calm, dear, deep, epic, feed, fine, free, gift, glow, heal, hear, help, hero, holy, hope, join, keen, kind, life, live, love, luck, mate, need, open, path, pour, pray, pure, real, rest, seep, soak, soul, swag, tact, team, true, wise, and well.

Chris is well. He is in good health both in mind and in body. He has recovered from his illness. If you want to say he is pretty well, well, that's all right. I am sure glad she didn't ask about the word *well*.

CHAPTER 41
FAITH THROUGH AFFLICTION

The secret things belong to the Lord our God, but the
things revealed belong to us and to our children forever,
that we may follow all the words of this law.
—*Deuteronomy 29:29*

Affliction is able to drown out every earthly voice ...
but the voice of eternity within a man it cannot drown.
When by the aid of affliction all irrelevant voices are
brought to silence, it can be heard, this voice within.
—*Søren Kierkegaard*

John Eldredge, in his popular book *Waking the Dead,* will offer our conclusion:

> Why are we enchanted by tales of transformation? The
> Phoenix rises from the ashes. Cinderella rises from the
> cinders to become a queen. The Ugly Duckling becomes
> a beautiful swan. The Cowardly Lion gets his courage,
> the Scarecrow his brains, and the Tin Woodman, a new
> heart. They are all transformed into the very thing they
> never thought they could be. Because that is the secret
> of the universe.[1]

What happened to you through your affliction? It is six years later, Chris, and you have experienced some pretty great things in that time. You have a granddaughter who calls you "Grandpa." You have improved your golf game and now shoot in the low 80s. You have held your wife countless nights and said, "I love you." You have seen the whales off the San Juan Islands, the grandeur of the Canadian Rockies, and the colors of New England in the fall, smiled and said "ahhhh." You've seen the pink moon. What beauty to behold! You are a good friend. You will talk to anyone who needs to know what to expect from this diagnosis. You have truly retired and own your day to do whatever you want. You have the cleanest garage of all the residents in the condo association (or so you'd like to believe). You have kissed your wife twice (2014 and 2017) in that time on the corner of Stockton and Fullerton on the course of the Chicago Marathon. You have worked on your tan. You drank a few awesome martinis made by Katia at Hawkshead Inn. You have identified the songs you want played at your funeral. You have reconciled with your son. You no longer have parents who are alive. You have reached the milestone of five years where all signs and symptoms of your cancer are undetectable. These years have been a gift to you and a gift to me.

Philip Yancy, in his book *Prayer: Does It Make Any Difference?*, says, "Faith during affliction matters more than healing from affliction."[2] God's purpose for each of us is to become fully alive. In the year before he was killed, German pastor and theologian Dietrich Bonhoeffer wrote to his friend: "May God lead us kindly through these times, but above all, may God lead us to himself." Dietrich carried his faith with him to the end. In his final moments, he exclaimed, "This is the end—for me the beginning of life."[3]

It doesn't matter, then, if you live or you die through whatever fight you are in. What matters is that you have invited Jesus into your heart, and you are with Him and He in you. Paul in his writings to the Galatians gets it right with: "What counts is whether we have been transformed into a new creation" (Galatians 6:15 NLT). We must deal with God if we want to be raised into newness of life. Have you changed into a new and different person? My prayer is that we all will get it right.

CHAPTER 42
COME HOME ALIVE

Heaven, the true meaning of the most precious word. Home.
—Mitch Albom

God cannot give us a happiness and peace apart from
Himself because it is not there. There is no such thing.
—C. S. Lewis

My childhood home is small-town middle America, with deep Christian values. The memories that play out are: sitting next to my childhood crush on the bus for out-of-town basketball games, telling my dad one July that Santa Claus was not real, riding my bike to summer school for a typing class so I would have something to keep me occupied and out of trouble during my summer break, getting a huge wad of gum stuck in my girlfriend's hair, singing with my class in the Christmas Eve program, freezing my hands and toes on a frigid walk home from school with my sister, sewing with my mom, doing laundry with my dad, having my hopes and dreams completely dashed when I didn't make the cheerleading squad, and swimming, swimming, and swimming some more at Evelyn and Vern Kettle's pool. During the long days and nights of Chris's journey, I was longing for my childhood home.

If you have resentment and bitterness about your childhood

memories, phone home[1] to your heavenly Father and ask Him to help you lose the weight of it. King David knew the Lord would be there, even though at times his parents were not. "Though my father and mother forsake me, the Lord will receive me" (Psalms 27:10). As parents, we do not always do the right thing, say the right thing, or make the right choice. Children forgive us. If you are carrying that extra weight, your heavenly Father has been waiting for you to phone home. He is there to hear your story and receive you, all of you. "Look to the Lord and His strength, seek His face always" (Psalm 105:4).

Mark Twain famously said, "A man who lives fully is prepared to die at any time." Life is something that you do. Life is for living. Live it today! A palliative care nurse from Australia wrote a book describing the top five regrets of the dying:

1. I wish I'd had the courage to live a life true to myself, not the life others expected of me.
2. I wish I hadn't worked so hard.
3. I wish I'd had the courage to express my feelings.
4. I wish I had stayed in touch with friends.
5. I wish I had let myself be happier.[2]

> Jesus said to her, "I am the resurrection and the life. He who believes in me will live, even though he dies; and whoever lives and believes in me will never die. Do you believe this?" (John 11:25)

At death you won't leave home—you'll go home. Earth is not our final home; we were all created for something much better. We can transcend death by keeping our eyes on and believing in our Risen Lord. So, whether you live or whether you die, you will come home alive.

Thank you, God, for teaching me to pray. Thank you for giving me the gift of intercession. Help me to use this gift each day to help those You have put into my path. May these prayers speak life into others' wounded souls. May these prayers save relationships. May these prayers heal others in their bodies, minds, and souls where there is the deepest hurt, the darkest illness, and the yet unknown assault. May these prayers save lives. May those lives in turn be thankful, and may your work on this earth multiply through them.

Rise up; this matter is in your hands. We will support you, so take courage and do it.

Ezra 10:4

PART 9

CALL TO ACTION

CHAPTER 43
CALL TO ACTION

If you want to change the world, pick up your pen and write.
—*Martin Luther*

In a gentle way, you can shake the world.
—*Mahatma Gandhi*

During the years of Chris's battle and beyond, John Eldredge has become a favorite author of mine. He writes, "Truth be told, you need to know the rest of the story if you want to understand just about anything in life ... none of it makes sense without a story."[1]

A growing number of middle-aged men and women are being diagnosed with HPV (human papillomavirus) cancer of the mouth, tonsils, or throat. It is one form of oropharyngeal cancer. This type of cancer caused by the HPV virus is being diagnosed in epidemic proportions in the United States and throughout the world as I finish this book.[2] This is what Chris was diagnosed with on November 22, 2013: HPV 16. Words I heard but did not understand at the time.

Nearly all sexually active people will get HPV at some time in their lives.[3] Many women, and now we are learning men as well, were likely exposed to cancer-causing HPV types in their teens and early twenties. Fifty percent of new HPV infections occur in fifteen- to twenty-four-year-olds.[4] Most people clear an HPV infection on their own within a year or two, but some people do not.[5] This was the case for Chris. He likely had been harboring this virus in his body for decades. Chris and I had just celebrated our thirtieth wedding anniversary a couple of months before his diagnosis. Another story I read was of a woman diagnosed with a tumor, also in her throat. She and her husband were married twenty-eight years at the time. I will ask you to not automatically judge that people who are diagnosed with this type of cancer deserve it and have it coming because of the numbers of different sex partners they have had. Yes, there are people who put themselves at greater risk for this diagnosis with the more sex partners they have had, but there are also couples who have been married for decades as we have been. What is important here to acknowledge is that whatever sexual encounters you have had in your lifetime stay with you for your lifetime. Each of us brought those into our marriage.

It takes many years before this virus becomes a cancer. HPV itself isn't cancer, but it can cause precancerous changes in our cells. What happens is that the virus tampers with our cells, and this can lead to cancer later.[6] Smoking and alcohol consumption further increase the risk that an HPV infection can and will become cancerous. The great news is that HPV positive tumors respond well to treatment.[7] The bad news is that the treatment for the disease is "insidious." Some might call it heavy-handed. I volunteer as a mentor to caregivers through a group called Imerman's Angels. In talking with one caregiver, I learned that all the teeth in a woman's mouth needed to be extracted prior to starting radiation treatment.

The number of people with this diagnosis, both males and females, is growing in epidemic proportions. Dr. Eric Moore, head and neck surgeon at the Mayo Clinic in Rochester, Minnesota, says, "This is a growing epidemic. It is a lump in the throat that won't go away. While most cancers are in a decline, this cancer is on the rise. The bottom line is that this is a tumor that is still increasing."[8]

HPV now causes about 70 percent of all oropharyngeal cancers in the United States. HPV head and neck cancers in the United States will surpass the number of cervical cancers by 2020. The majority of HPV infection is heterosexual. It is a "small virus with big consequences."[9]

The public is largely unaware of this growing epidemic. The Lord would not let me alone. Therefore, I believe that I have been called to tell this story. "There's a social stigma associated with HPV related head and neck cancer, and it's something that patients feel shy or uncomfortable talking about to their peers. And this may be one of the barriers that may be preventing a full awareness of this disease," states Dr. Sara Pai, associate professor at Johns Hopkins School of Medicine, Department of Otolaryngology—Head and Neck Surgery.[10] This social stigma prevents progress, and we must get over it. We must talk about it. More conversations will help break down the unease associated with the disease and speed efforts to find gentler treatments to reduce the long-term side effects.

In the 1920s, Dr. George Papanicolaou developed a test that can discover cancer from a smear in the uterine cervix. Many women know this as the PAP smear or PAP test. It was not until the 1940s that it became a standard test for detecting cervical cancer in women.[11] The PAP test has been applauded as the most successful cancer screening technique in history. Dr. Papanicolaou can be found on the list of Science Heroes, as it is believed that this simple test has saved over six million lives since World War II.[12]

What is a bit surprising to me is that many people do not even know what a PAP smear or PAP test is for. It is a way to detect abnormal cervical cells and early cervical cancer. Nearly all cases of cervical cancer are HPV related.[13] This screening is an essential part of a woman's routine health care. I have received a PAP smear annually, and more recently according to plan guidelines, since age twenty-one. The guidelines have loosened recently, and now women should have a PAP smear every three years. And even though we have a silver bullet here for women, in 2012 there were 12,170 new cases of cervical cancer diagnosed in the United States and 4,220 of those women would die. However, women whose cervical cancers were found by a PAP test had a 92 percent cure rate.[14] PAP smears find cancers at an earlier and more treatable stage.

But what about the men? Currently there is no standard or routine screening to test for unusual cell growth in the oral cavity, pharyngeal, and laryngeal areas.[15] Why is there currently no test or screening for the throat and mouth area? I want to know why. Here is the most widely used cancer screening method in the world, which has saved countless lives, but we can't find a way to make it transferrable to men and women, potentially to screen the oral and throat cavity?

To my great surprise and delight, the last time I visited our dentist, it appeared that new protocols were in place to assist in detecting early warning signs for oral cavity cancer. As a standard practice, my hygienist asked me several questions about having a sore throat. I wanted to learn if these questions and additional physical examinations were triggered by revised or updated protocols. Doug Bleyenburg, DDS, said, "Yes, there is greater awareness of the severity of throat cancer. We want to be more vigilant and thorough in observing signs of lumps and sores through our visual and tactile examinations."

Our regular dentist is a partner in the fight against oral cancer and should check for suspicious spots and feel for lumps in and around the mouth. It is important for you to tell your dentist if you experience any sores that bleed easily, or do not heal; or any thick, hard spots or lumps, and a sore throat that does not go away.[16]

In a conversation with another local dentist regarding oral cavity cancers, he said, "As dentists, we are aware of our role as cotreaters and partners in our patients' health. We can get into bad habits, but now we are more conscientious about anything we observe. Today, I palpate the neck of my patients."

Start a conversation and continue to ask questions. We need to educate primary care physicians and dental providers regarding this epidemic that is growing in our communities.

The breakthrough is that we do have an HPV vaccine for young people. It is now a vaccine that is part of the routine childhood schedule. This vaccine, however, cannot treat an existing HPV infection.[17] In October 2016 the guidelines were loosened. They include that all adolescents and teens ages nine to fourteen should receive two doses at least six months apart. Teens who receive the vaccine later should continue to receive three doses.[18] I would like to propose that it become a school enrollment requirement. This will need to be decided state by state. Widespread immunization for HPV could reduce the impact not only in girls but boys as well. Dr. Moore continues, "Vaccine is a sure-fire way to drop the incidence in the future."[19]

Pamela Tom, founder of HPVANDME, a nonprofit organization dedicated to providing education about HPV prevention and HPV-related oropharyngeal cancer, states: "Every doctor who I have spoken with agrees that if HPV vaccination rates increase to near 100 percent, we can nearly eradicate all HPV-related cancers in a few generations. Now that's something to talk about."[20]

But this still leaves the group in the middle, like my children. Together we have three sons, ages forty-two, forty-five, and forty-nine. The vaccine was introduced in 2006. We have two generations that are at risk today—mine and my children's. In 2013, Tom Frieden, the director of the CDC (Centers for Disease Control) shared results of a study that showed that "the prevalence of HPV has decreased by 56 percent among teenagers since the vaccine was introduced in 2006. This is a wake-up call to our nation to protect the next generation." Lauri Markowitz, the lead on the study, indicated: "This decline is encouraging given the substantial health and economic burden of HPV-associated disease."[21] But sadly, as of October 2017, only 49 percent of 13- to 17-year-old boys and girls are receiving this vaccine. In 2018 it was 51 percent.[22] We are making progress, and the numbers continue to increase for those that are vaccinated, but it still leaves half of that population group exposed. This must change.

There's a pharmacy in our town that I frequent—Paul's Pharmacy. While writing this book, I came to the front door of the store, and to my shock and surprise, a large poster said, "If there were a vaccine against cancer, wouldn't you get it for your kids?"

Vaccines are not for everyone, and side effects need to be investigated and understood for your unique situation. But after what we have gone through, absolutely, 100 percent I would.

And now you know the story. None of it makes sense without the story.

AFTERWORD
BECAUSE OF THE VIRUS

Failure is not fatal, but failure to change might be.
—*John Wooden*

Here is the world. Beautiful and terrible
things will happen. Do not be afraid.
—*Frederick Buechner*

Easter Sunday 2020. We are positioned on our bar stools at the breakfast counter of our kitchen looking into the screen of a laptop computer. We look at each other and proclaim, "He is risen; He is risen indeed!" There is only the sound of our two voices. But then, we say it again louder: "He is risen, He is risen indeed!"

Because of the coronavirus, churches are closed, and we are not able to celebrate with others the glorious resurrection of Jesus Christ. Because of the virus, our offices are closed. Because of the virus, millions around the world are out of work. There are long lines of people waiting to find the food they will need for their families, for just today. Then, what will they do tomorrow? Because of the virus, we are told to stay at home. Here we are today worshipping our risen Lord alone but, magnificently, together.

Viruses cause many human diseases. But now we painfully know that viruses are deadly. *Silent killer. Invisible enemy.* Viruses destroy lives.

We also know that viruses, such as the human papilloma virus, can lead to cancer, and sadly, death.

The common cold is a virus. Different types of flus are viruses. Polio, rabies, Ebola, SARS, measles, mumps, chicken pox, and shingles, all these are viruses.[1] We have a new perspective on the word "virus" post-2019. People jokingly now say, "Hindsight is 2020." Scientists are very concerned about rare viruses that spread from animals to people. These can create a pandemic. All of us are experiencing the consequences of the pandemic caused by the coronavirus.

In the 1980s, polio crippled an estimated 350,000 children globally. By 2018 that number was down to a total of just thirty-three reported cases.[2] What changed the history of polio forever was the development of a vaccine against the disease.

There is no cure for a virus, but a vaccination can prevent it from spreading. So, we wait for that vaccine to be developed to eradicate COVID-19—the coronavirus.

There is no wait for the vaccine for HPV; we have it. It is available now. Amid the crisis and upheaval—the magnitude of a pandemic—it is easy to lose sight of the consequences and implications of an epidemic.

DISCLAIMER PAGE

We have yet to find a universal cure for cancer. This is our story. This is the way we chose to cope, manage, and live each day from diagnosis through continued recovery today. This is in no way a treatment plan, or a guarantee of healing and survival.

Not all throat and oral cavity cancers are caused by the HPV virus. There is no inference in this book of that nature.

This book is not intended as a substitute for the medical advice of physicians. The reader should regularly consult a physician in matters relating to his/her health and particularly with respect to any symptoms that may require diagnosis or medical attention.

The events are described from journals, time lines, and text messages. Some of the events and their chronological order have been moved to minimize confusion.

Some names and identifying details have been changed to protect the privacy of individuals.

ACKNOWLEDGMENTS

Lou Kasischke: Thank you for providing the words and the inspiration.

Henri Paterson: I miss you. Thank you for giving me the foundation—the power is in the knowing.

Donna Mantey: Thank you for always being there—morning, noon, and night. Thank you for approaching the throne.

Kathy Kolbe: Thank you for giving me your truths and your wisdom.

Kelli Barendse: Thank you for opening the box of a thousand puzzle pieces that were all white and helping me see the shapes and sizes. You were exactly the right person at the right time in the right role.

Monica Gravenhof: Thank you for keeping the business going when my thoughts, emotions, and actions were required elsewhere. We couldn't have made it through without you.

My ministry friends: Thank you for praying me through. It's a book!

Karl and Betty Mantey, my parents: Thank you for living a full life following Jesus and providing an example of Christian behavior and loving discipline in our home.

Ara and Geoff Crittenden: Without you, the stories of my life would not exist.

Cast of Characters: Bill, Dave, John, Tom, Mike, Don, Frank, Paul, Cal, Wally, Wayne, Jeanine, and various others who sat around the table at one point or another to "solve the world's problems one cup at a time." Thank you for your support and encouragement during those uncertain and scary times.

Monty Mantey, Morris Mantey, and Monica Morris: Family is the feeling that your heart is home again. Thank you for making our family the best on earth that any baby sister could ever want to be a part of.

Caroline Crittenden: As you began to learn and use words, your expression, "Grandma, have a help," had a dual meaning, not only of "I need your help," but also of "I want to help you." Learning to discern is what helping is all about. Pretty profound.

Early readers: Chris Martin, Monica Morris, Donna Mantey, Monica Gravenhof, Ara Crittenden, Geoff Crittenden, Dianne Bierma, Dave VanOpstall, Lyndsey Tym, and Gwen Auwerda. I appreciated the many words of encouragement and suggestions for improvement that will always be *just between you and me.*

CVS Pharmacy staff: You were our dedicated partners in care. Thank you for showing concern and compassion when we were walking in darkness and unsure of where the next step would lead.

Chris Martin: I'd do it all again with you, but let's choose a different adventure next time, okay?

NOTES

Inspiration

1   Louis W. Kasischke and Jane Cardinal, *After the Wind: 1996 Everest Tragedy—One Survivor's Story*, (Good Hart, 2014).

Running Renegade

1   John Eldredge, "Waking the Dead" in *The Ransomed Heart: A Collection of Devotional Readings* (Thomas Nelson, 2005), 122.
2   Rick Warren, *The Purpose-Driven Life: What on Earth Am I Here For?* (Zondervan, 2002), 57.
3   Toby Mac, "Speak Life," *Eye on It,* ForeFront, 2012.
4   "Lifetime Risk of Developing or Dying from Cancer," American Cancer Society, accessed January 9, 2020, www.cancer.org/cancer/cancer-basics/lifetime-probability-of-developing-or-dying-from-cancer.html.
5   "Cancer Facts & Figures 2020," American Cancer Society, accessed January 10, 2020, www.cancer.org/research/cancer-facts-statistics/all-cancer-facts-figures/cancer-facts-figures-2020.html.
6   Bruce Grierson, *What Makes Olga Run?: The Mystery of the 90-Something Track Star and What She Can Teach Us About Living Longer, Happier Lives* (St. Martin's Griffin, 2015), 18.
7   Warren, *Purpose-Driven Life*, 301.
8   John Eldredge, *Moving Mountains: Praying with Passion, Confidence, and Authority* (Thomas Nelson, 2017), 224–25.

Diagnosis

1   Gary Gillette, "Willie Hernandez." Willie Hernandez | Society for American Baseball Research, accessed January 19, 2020, sabr.org/bioproj/person/c8f40717.

Ticking Time Bomb

1   *Castle,* season 5, episode 22, "Still," directed by Bill Roe, written by Rob Hanning, performed by Nathan Fillion, Stana Katic, Susan Sullivan, and Jon Huertas, aired April 29, 2013, in broadcast syndication, ABC Studios, 2013, DVD.

Light for the Way They Should Take

1   "Trust." Dictionary.com, accessed January 20, 2020, www.dictionary.com/browse/trust.
2   *Sully,* directed by Clint Eastwood (Burbank, CA: Warner Home Video, 2016), DVD.
3   Sarah Young, *Jesus Calling: Enjoying Peace in His Presence* (Thomas Nelson, 2004), 28.
4   "Cancer Staging," National Cancer Institute, accessed January 26, 2020, www.cancer.gov/about-cancer/diagnosis-staging/staging.
5   Kulbhushaan Raghuvanshi, "Stage 4 Throat Cancer Prognosis." Health Hearty, accessed January 23, 2020, healthhearty.com/stage4-throat-cancer-prognosis.

Do Not Be Afraid

1   Hurricane Matthew was a Category 5 hurricane that affected the Caribbean (primarily the islands of Hispaniola, Cuba, and the Bahamas) and the Southeastern United States. At its peak, it had winds up to 165 miles per hour. It was responsible for 585 deaths, making it the deadliest Atlantic hurricane since 2005.
Stacy R. Stewart, Rep. *Hurricane Matthew,* April 7, 2017. https://www.nhc.noaa.gov/data/tcr/AL142016_Matthew.pdf.

Phone Home

1   *E.T. the Extra-Terrestrial,* directed by Steven Spielberg (1982; Universal City, CA: Universal Studios, 2002), DVD.

The Gift of Presence

1   Joe E. Pennel, *The Gift of Presence: A Guide to Helping Those Who Suffer* (Abingdon Press, 2009), 10, 23.
2   Sherry Turkle, *Alone Together: Why We Expect More from Technology and Less from Each Other* (Basic Books, 2011).

3 Pennel, *Gift of Presence*, 87.

4 Max Lucado, *Fearless: Imagine Your Life Without Fear* (Thomas Nelson, 2009).

5 Stormie Omartian, *Just Enough Light for the Step I'm On: Trusting God in the Tough Times* (Harvest House, 2002).

Prayer

1 Bruce L. Bugbee and Don Cousins. *Network Participant's Guide* (Zondervan, 2004), 87.

2 Bugbee and Cousins, Network Participant's Guide, 87.

3 Young, *Jesus Calling*.

4 Sarah Young, *Jesus Today: Experience Hope Through His Presence* (Thomas Nelson, 2012).

5 Peter Scazzero, *Daily Office—Remembering God's Presence Throughout the Day: Begin the Journey* (Willow Creek Association, 2008).

6 Stormie Omartian, *The Power of a Praying Life Book of Prayers: Finding the Freedom, Wholeness, and True Success God Has for You* (Harvest House, 2010).

7 *NIV Couples' Devotional Bible* (Zondervan, 1994).

8 Tom Brokaw, *A Lucky Life Interrupted: A Memoir of Hope* (Random House, 2015), 156–57.

9 Pennel, *Gift of Presence*, 62.

10 Philip Yancey, *Prayer: Does It Make Any Difference?* 2nd ed. (Hodder, 2008), 254.

11 R. T. Kendall, *The Lord's Prayer* (Hodder & Stoughton, 2011), 101, 104.

12 Mitch Albom, *Have a Little Faith: A True Story* (Hachette Books, 2009), 82.

13 Ed Strauss, *The Top 100 Prayers of the Bible* (Barbour, 2016), 119.

14 Yancey, *Prayer: Does It Make Any Difference?*, 58.

15 Henry Blackaby and Norman Blackaby, *Experiencing Prayer with Jesus: The Power of His Presence and Example* (Crown, 2005), 29.

16 Lucado, *Fearless: Imagine Your Life Without Fear.*

17 Yancey, *Prayer: Does It Make Any Difference?*, 35.

Prayer Focus

1 Blackaby and Blackaby, *Experiencing Prayer with Jesus,* 94.

2 Blackaby and Blackaby, Experiencing Prayer, 132.

3 Yancey, *Prayer: Does It Make Any Difference?*, 153.

4 Dutch Sheets, *Intercessory Prayer: How God Can Use Your Prayers to Move Heaven and Earth* (Baker Books, 1996), 198, 211.

5 Charles R. Swindoll, *Living the Proverbs: Insights for the Daily Grind* (Worthy Books, 2012), 47–48.

We Believe

1   Yancey, *Prayer: Does It Make Any Difference?*, 236.

2   "P.J Fleck." University of Minnesota Athletics, accessed February 2, 2020, gophersports.com/sports/football/roster/coaches/p-j-fleck/1918.

3   Western Michigan Bronco Athletics. "Coach Fleck Video Series: Row the Boat," YouTube, May 29, 2013, video, 9:19, https://www.youtube.com/watch?v=PaAnElqNNrQ.

4   Omartian, *Just Enough Light for the Step I'm On,* 40.

5   Mark Cartwright, "Centurion," Ancient History Encyclopedia, July 4, 2014, www.ancient.eu/Centurion/.

6   Strauss, *Top 100 Prayers of the Bible,* 148.

7   Strauss, 152.

8   Strauss, 153.

9   Strauss, 156.

You Are Not a Doctor

1   "9.5 Fasting Blood Sugar Levels Non Diabetic," Diabetes Daily Forums, April 23, 2018, www.diabetesdaily.com/forum/threads/9-5-fasting-blood-sugar-levels-non-diabetic.116091/.

Hospital

1   Mayo Clinic Staff, "Diabetic Coma," Mayo Clinic, last modified June 26, 2020, www.mayoclinic.org/diseases-conditions/diabetic-coma/symptoms-causes/syc-20371475.

Thriving to Heal

1   "What Is Cancer? Common Forms and Oncology Treatment Options," Cancer Treatment Centers of America, accessed January 28, 2020, www.cancercenter.com/what-is-cancer.

2   Gretchen Rubin, *The Happiness Project* (HarperCollins, 2009), 11, 288.

3   Kathy Kolbe and David Kolbe, "Management by Instinct Leads the Way to Change," Kolbe Corp., last modified 2002, https://static1.squarespace.com/static/5ae52b0fec4eb74b617ae193/t/5af8dc7470a6ad26b067c809/1526258804748/InsightSC-Management+by+Instinct+Leads.pdf.

4   William James, "What is an Instinct?" *Scribner's Magazine*, March 1887, 355.

5   "What Is Stress?" American Institute of Stress, accessed February 11, 2020, www.stress.org/daily-life.

6   "America's #1 Health Problem," American Institute of Stress, January 4, 2017, www.stress.org/americas-1-health-problem.

7   Yancey, *Prayer: Does It Make Any Difference?*, 254.

Kolbe Is a Breakthrough

1   Bill Taylor, "What Breaking the 4-Minute Mile Taught Us About the Limits of Conventional Thinking," Harvard Business Review, March 9, 2018, hbr.org/2018/03/what-breaking-the-4-minute-mile-taught-us-about-the-limits-of-conventional-thinking.

2   Andrew Keh, "Eliud Kipchoge Breaks Two-Hour Marathon Barrier," *New York Times*, October 12, 2019, www.nytimes.com/2019/10/12/sports/eliud-kipchoge-marathon-record.html.

3   "Home of the Kolbe A™ Index," Kolbe.com | Home of the Kolbe A™ Index, Kolbe Corp, 2020, www.kolbe.com/.

4   Tony DuFrene, "Two Boats and a Helicopter. Thoughts on Stress Management," *Psychology Today,* Sussex, May 4, 2009, https://www.psychologytoday.com/us/blog/fumbling-change/200905/two-boats-and-helicopter-thoughts-stress-management.

5   Gary Chapman, *The Five Love Languages: How to Express Heartfelt Commitment to Your Mate* (Northfield, 1992), 10.

Acting on What You Know

1   Timothy E. Paterick MD, *Invest in Yourself: A Cardiologist's Narrative for Heart Health* (CreateSpace Independent Publishing Platform, 2014), 29.

Know Your Modus Operandi (MO)

1   Marie Kondo, *The Life-Changing Magic of Tidying Up: The Japanese Art of Decluttering and Organizing* (Ten Speed Press, 2014).

2   Grierson, *What Makes Olga Run?*, 225.

3   T. D. Jakes, *Woman, Thou Art Loosed!: Healing the Wounds of the Past* (Destiny Image, 2011), 123.

4   Jakes, 125–26.

5   Marcus Buckingham, *The One Thing You Need to Know: … About Great Managing, Great Leading and Sustained Individual Success* (Simon and Schuster, 2008), 21–22.

Who Is in Your Boat?

1 "Life of Pi: Book Summary," CliffsNotes, Houghton Mifflin Harcourt, accessed March 6, 2020, www.cliffsnotes.com/literature/l/life-of-pi/book-summary.

2 Harlan Coben, *Run Away* (Grand Central, 2019), 140.

3 Stormie Omartian, *Power of a Praying Wife* (Kingsway, 1997), 31.

4 Omartian, 46.

5 Emerson Eggerichs, *Love and Respect: The Love She Most Desires; The Respect He Desperately Needs* (Integrity, 2004), 35.

In Relationship

1 Charles R. Swindoll, *Growing Deep in the Christian Life* (Zondervan, 1995), 199.

2 "Peace (in the Bible)," New Catholic Encyclopedia, Encyclopedia.com, January 25, 2020, www.encyclopedia.com/religion/encyclopedias-almanacs-transcripts-and-maps/peace-bible.

3 Albom, *Have a Little Faith,* 221.

4 T. D. Jakes, *The Great Investment: Faith, Family, and Finance* (Putnam's Sons, 2000), 81.

5 Thomas L. Friedman, *Thank You for Being Late: An Optimist's Guide to Thriving in the Age of Accelerations* (Farrar, Straus, and Giroux, 2016), 354.

Do Not Die of Caregiving

1 "Portrait of an ESFJ," The Personality Page, BSM Consulting, accessed March 10, 2020, www.personalitypage.com/html/ESFJ.html.

2 Hurricane Harvey was a category 4 hurricane that primarily affected southeastern Texas. It stalled near the Texas coast for four days, which resulted in historic rainfall and flooding (sixty-plus inches in some locations.) It is the second costliest hurricane for the United States and resulted in sixty-eight deaths. Eric S. Blake and David A. Zelinsky, Rep. *Hurricane Harvey*, May 9, 2018. https://www.nhc.noaa.gov/data/tcr/AL092017_Harvey.pdf.

3 Grierson, *What Makes Olga Run?,* 170–71.

Decision Fatigue

1 John Tierney and Roy F. Baumeister, *Willpower: Rediscovering the Greatest Human Strength* (Penguin Books, 2011), 98-99, 156.

2 Jay Papasan and James Clear, "Habits, Not Goals, Will Bring You Success," Next Big Idea Club, August 10, 2017, heleo.com/conversation-habits-not-goals-will-bring-you-success/15837/.

3   Kathy Kolbe, *Powered by Instinct: 5 Rules for Trusting Your Gut* (Monumentus Press, 2004), 4.

This Could Go Either Way

1   "Home: Tulip Time." Tulip Time, May 2–10, 2020, Holland, MI, Tulip Time Festival, accessed March 12, 2020, www.tuliptime.com/.

Just Between You and Me

1   Oswald Chambers, "October 11: After God's Silence—What?" in *My Utmost for His Highest* (Dodd, Mead, 1935), 296–97.

I Run to Hear

1   Queen, "We Are the Champions," recorded 1977, track 2 on *News of the World,* Elektra, compact disc.
2   American Cancer Society, "Lifetime Risk of Developing or Dying from Cancer."

What I've Learned about Cancer

1   Siddhartha Mukherjee, *The Emperor of All Maladies: A Biography of Cancer* (Scribner, 2010), 329.
2   "Cancer Statistics," National Cancer Institute, April 27, 2018, www.cancer.gov/about-cancer/understanding/statistics.
3   "Cancer Facts & Figures 2018." American Cancer Society, 2018, www.cancer.org/content/dam/cancer-org/research/cancer-facts-and-statistics/annual-cancer-facts-and-figures/2018/cancer-facts-and-figures-2018.pdf.
4   Mike Garten, "Disease Detection: Are You up to Date on Your Screenings?" *Good Housekeeping*, October 2019, 78.
5   Heather Carlson Kehren, "Mayo Researchers Find 'Unacceptable Low' Cervical Cancer Screening Rates," Mayo Clinic, January 7, 2019, newsnetwork.mayoclinic.org/discussion/mayo-researchers-find-unacceptable-low-cervical-cancer-screening-rates/.
6   Kellie Bramlet Blackburn, "Diabetes and Cancer: What You Should Know," MD Anderson Cancer Center, May 2017, www.mdanderson.org/publications/focused-on-health/Diabetes-and-cancer.h26Z1591413.html.
7   Erika Gebel, "Diabetes and Cancer: What's the Connection?" Diabetes Forecast, October 2012, www.diabetesforecast.org/2012/oct/diabetes-and-cancer-what-s-the-connection.html.

8   Emily Jane Gallagher and Derek LeRoith, "Obesity and Diabetes: The Increased Risk of Cancer and Cancer-Related Mortality," *Physiological Reviews* 95, no. 3 (July 1, 2015) 727–48, journals.physiology.org/doi/full/10.1152/physrev.00030.2014.

9   Kellie Bramlet Blackburn, "How to Manage Diabetes and Cancer Treatment," MD Anderson Cancer Center, May 3, 2017, www.mdanderson.org/publications/cancerwise/how-to-manage-diabetes-and-cancer-treatment.h00-159145245.html.

10   Mukherjee, *The Emperor of All Maladies: A Biography of Cancer.*

11   "Common Cancer Myths and Misconceptions," National Cancer Institute, August 22, 2018, www.cancer.gov/about-cancer/causes-prevention/risk/myths.

12   Peggy Hesketh, *Telling the Bees* (G. P. Putnam's Sons, 2013).

13   Cancer Treatment Centers of America, "What Is Cancer? Common Forms and Oncology Treatment Options."

Be Grateful and Thankful

1   Ann Voskamp, *One Thousand Gifts: A Dare to Live Fully Right Where You Are* (Zondervan, 2011), 33–34.

2   Voskamp, 37.

3   Ed Strauss, *Top 100 Prayers of the Bible*, 169–70.

4   Voskamp, *One Thousand Gifts,* 39.

Do You Believe in Miracles?

1   Referring to the "miracle on ice" that occurred when the United States hockey team played their Olympic match against the highly favored, four-time defending gold medalists, the Soviet Union. The United States would go on to beat Finland, and ultimately win the gold medal, their first in twenty years and second overall. "THE 1980 U.S. OLYMPIC TEAM," US Hockey Hall of Fame, accessed March 6, 2020, https://www.ushockeyhalloffame.com/page/show/831562-the-1980-u-s-olympic-team.

2   Sheets, *Intercessory Prayer,* 100.

3   Thomas Moore, "Jesus and the Soul of the Gospels" in *Writing in the Sand* (Hay House, 2009), 34–35.

4   Sarah Young, "December 21," in *Jesus Calling*, 372.

Time Line of a Miracle

1   The V Foundation for Cancer Research, "Jim's 1993 ESPY Speech," YouTube, September 28, 2008, video, 11:14, https://www.youtube.com/watch?v =HuoVM9nm42E.

The Miracle of New Life

1   "Expect," Lexico, Oxford Dictionary, last modified 2020, www.lexico.com/ en/definition/expect.

The Miracle of a Healing Practice

1   Michael Devitt, "Acupuncture of Dry Mouth," *Acupuncture Today* 1, no. 11 (November 2000), www.acupuncturetoday.com/mpacms/at/article. php?id=27653.

The Miracle of Love

1   Sue Miller, *The Senator's Wife* (Bloomsbury, 2008), 188.
2   Nicholas Sparks, *The Best of Me* (Grand Central, 2011), 167, 288.
3   Timothy Keller, *The Meaning of Marriage: Facing the Complexities of Marriage with the Wisdom of God* (John Murray Press, 2011), 101.

Chicago Marathon 2017

1   Referring to the famous line sports commentator Howard Cosell used during a heavyweight match between Joe Frazier and George Foreman. The fight, dubbed "The Sunshine Showdown," was one between two undefeated punchers. Frazier, the then undisputed heavyweight champion, was handily beaten in less than two rounds.
James Slater, "45 Years Ago Today: 'Down Goes Frazier! Down Goes Frazier!,'" Boxing News 24/7, East Side Boxing, January 22, 2018, https:// www.boxing247.com/boxing-news/45-years-ago-today-down-goes-frazier-down-goes-frazier/88647.
2   *The Silence of the Lambs*, directed by Jonathan Demme (1992; Los Angeles, CA: Orion Pictures, 2001), DVD.
3   Galen Rupp is an American long-distance runner. He competed in the 2012 Olympics where he earned the silver medal for the ten thousand meters and the 2016 Olympics where he earned the bronze medal for the marathon

event. He placed first at the 2017 and 2018 Chicago Marathons. "World Athletics: Galen RUPP: Profile," World Athletics, accessed March 18, 2020, https://worldathletics.org/athletes/united-states/galen-rupp-14250207.

4   Abraham Lincoln, "Second Inaugural Address," March 4, 1865, Capitol, Washington DC, address.

5   Refers to previous winners of the Chicago Marathon. Greg Meyer was the last American-born runner to win the Chicago Marathon (1982) before Galen Rupp in 2017. Joan Benoit-Samuelson had the fastest time for an American woman at the Chicago Marathon during her win in 1985. Paula Radcliffe won the event in 2002.

6   Roy Lessin, *From God's Heart to Yours* (David C. Cook, 2001), 69.

7   *Cool Runnings*, directed by Jon Turteltaub, 1993; Burbank, CA: Buena Vista Pictures, 1999), DVD.

Pretty Well

1   "Well." Lexico, Oxford Dictionary, last modified 2020, https://www.lexico.com/en/definition/well.

Faith through Affliction

1   Eldredge, John, *Waking the Dead: The Glory of a Heart Fully Alive* (Thomas Nelson, 2006), 56–57.

2   Yancey, *Prayer: Does It Make Any Difference?*, 325.

3   Abram K. J., "Bonhoeffer's Last Words, Before He Was Hanged (69 Years Ago Tomorrow)," *Words on the Word* (blog), April 8, 2014, abramkj.com/2014/04/08/bonhoeffers-last-words-before-he-was-hanged-69-years-ago-tomorrow/.

Come Home Alive

1   Spielberg, *E.T. the Extra-Terrestrial.*

2   Bronnie Ware, *The Top Five Regrets of the Dying: A Life Transformed by the Dearly Departing* (Hay House, 2011).

Call to Action

1   Eldredge, "Life is a Story, Epic" in *The Ransomed Heart*, 2–4.

2   Maggie Fox, "A Silent Epidemic of Cancer Is Spreading among Men." NBCNews.com, October 17, 2017, www.nbcnews.com/health/health-news/silent-epidemic-cancer-spreading-among-men-n811466.

3 "STD Facts—HPV and Men," Centers for Disease Control and Prevention, December 28, 2016, www.cdc.gov/std/hpv/stdfact-hpv-and-men.htm.

4 Lauri E. Markowitz et al., "Human Papillomavirus Vaccination: Recommendations of the Advisory Committee on Immunization Practices (ACIP)," Centers for Disease Control and Prevention, August 29, 2014, www.cdc.gov/mmwr/preview/mmwrhtml/rr6305a1.htm.

5 Katherine Harmon, "HPV-Positive Cancers Spreading among the Middle-Aged," *Scientific American*, November 2, 2010, www.scientificamerican.com/article/sex-spreads-hpv-cancers/.

6 "Basic Information about HPV and Cancer," Centers for Disease Control and Prevention, August 22, 2018, www.cdc.gov/cancer/hpv/basic_info/index.htm.

7 Mayo Clinic, "HPV-related throat cancer: Mayo Clinic Radio," YouTube, August 19, 2018, video, 9:33, https://www.youtube.com/watch?v=YnkDsJJ_blI.

8 Mayo Clinic, "HPV Head and Neck Cancers: Mayo Clinic Radio," YouTube, July 26, 2019, video, 10:16, https://www.youtube.com/watch?v=MRj7LOcs3K0.

9 "HPV Awareness and Education - HPVANDME: A Non-Profit Organization," HPVANDME, last modified 2020, hpvandme.org/.

10 HPVANDME.ORG. "HPV Throat Cancer: Partners and the Social Stigma" YouTube, June 8, 2013, video, 1:40, https://www.youtube.com/watch?v=uIpx_2hHIVo.

11 Siang Yong Tan and Yvonne Tatsumura, "George Papanicolaou (1883–1962): Discoverer of the Pap Smear," *Singapore Medical Journal* (October 2015) doi:10.11622/smedj.2015155.

12 Tim Anderson, "Georgios Papanikolaou," Science Heroes, accessed March 29, 2020, scienceheroes.com/index.php?option=com_content&view=article&id=183&Itemid=182.

13 Emma Smith, "HPV: The Whole Story, Warts and All." Cancer Research UK, September 16, 2014, scienceblog.cancerresearchuk.org/2014/09/16/hpv-the-whole-story-warts-and-all/.

14 Denise Mann, "Study Reaffirms That Pap Tests Save Lives," WebMD, March 1, 2012, www.webmd.com/women/news/20120301/study-reaffirms-pap-tests-save-lives.

15 HPV and Me, "HPV Awareness and Education."

16 "Early Signs of Oral Cancer," Cigna Dental Health, October 2016, www.cigna.com/individuals-families/health-wellness/early-signs-oral-cancer.

17 Carole Fakhry and Gypsyamber D'Souza, "Discussing the Diagnosis of HPV-OSCC: Common Questions and Answers." *Oral Oncology*, July 19, 2013, https://www.ncbi.nlm.nih.gov/pmc/articles/PMC4264664/.

18 "The HPV Vaccine - HPVANDME: A Non-Profit Organization." HPVANDME, accessed March 30, 2020, hpvandme.org/the-hpv-vaccine/.

19 Mayo Clinic, "HPV Head and Neck Cancers: Mayo Clinic Radio."

20 Pamela Tom, "HPV: This Common Virus Needs a Voice—HPVANDME: A Non-Profit Organization," HPVANDME, March 4, 2019, hpvandme.org/hpv-this-common-virus-needs-a-voice/.

21 "New Study Shows HPV Vaccine Helping Lower HPV Infection Rates in Teen Girls," Centers for Disease Control and Prevention, June 19, 2013, www.cdc.gov/media/releases/2013/p0619-hpv-vaccinations.html.

22 Melissa Jenco, "CDC: Teens' HPV Vaccination Rates Improve Slightly," American Academy of Pediatrics, August 22, 2019, www.aappublications.org/news/2019/08/22/teenvaccination082219.

Afterword

1 Peter Crosta, "What to Know about Viruses," *Medical News Today*, May 30, 2017, www.medicalnewstoday.com/articles/158179.

"Poliomyelitis," World Health Organization, July 22, 2019, www.who.int/news-room/fact-sheets/detail/poliomyelitis.

RECOMMENDED READING

Prayer:

John Eldredge, *Moving Mountains: Praying with Passion, Confidence, and Authority* (Thomas Nelson, 2017).

Dutch Sheets, *Intercessory Prayer: How God Can Use Your Prayers to Move Heaven and Earth* (Baker Books, 1996).

Ed Strauss, *The Top 100 Prayers of the Bible* (Barbour, 2016).

Philip Yancey, *Prayer: Does It Make Any Difference?* 2nd ed. (Hodder, 2008).

Devotional:

John Eldredge, *The Ransomed Heart: A Collection of Devotional Readings* (Thomas Nelson, 2005).

Sarah Young, *Jesus Calling: Enjoying Peace in His Presence* (Thomas Nelson, 2004).

Couples:

Emerson Eggerichs, *Love and Respect: The Love She Most Desires; The Respect He Desperately Needs* (Integrity, 2004).

Timothy Keller, *The Meaning of Marriage: Facing the Complexities of Marriage with the Wisdom of God* (John Murray Press, 2011).

Self-Care:

Timothy E. Paterick, *Invest in Yourself: A Cardiologist's Narrative for Heart Health* (CreateSpace Independent Publishing Platform, 2014).

Gretchen Rubin, *Better Than Before: What I Learned About Making and Breaking Habits—to Sleep More, Quit Sugar, Procrastinate Less, and Generally Build a Happier Life* (Broadway Books, 2015).

Gretchen Rubin, *The Happiness Project* (HarperCollins, 2009).

Wisdom:

Mitch Albom, *Have a Little Faith: A True Story* (Hachette Books, 2009).

Henry T. Blackaby et al., *Experiencing God: Knowing and Doing the Will of God, Revised and Expanded* (B&H Books, 2008).

Bruce L Bugbee and Don Cousins, *Network Participant's Guide* (Zondervan, 2004).

Charles Duhigg, *The Power of Habit: Why We Do What We Do in Life and Business* (Random House, 2012).

A. J. Gregory, *Silent Savior: Daring to Believe He's Still There* (Revell, 2009).

Bruce Grierson, *What Makes Olga Run?: The Mystery of the 90-Something Track Star and What She Can Teach Us About Living Longer, Happier Lives* (St. Martin's Griffin, 2015).

T. D. Jakes, *Life Overflowing, 6-in-1: 6 Pillars for Abundant Living* (Bethany House, 2010).

T. D. Jakes, *The Lady, Her Lover, and Her Lord* (Berkley, 2000).

T. D. Jakes, *Woman, Thou Art Loosed!: Healing the Wounds of the Past* (Destiny Image, 2011).

Thomas Moore, "Jesus and the Soul of the Gospels," in *Writing in the Sand* (Hay House, 2009).

John Tierney and Roy F. Baumeister, *Willpower: Rediscovering the Greatest Human Strength* (Penguin Books, 2011).

Ann Voskamp, *One Thousand Gifts: A Dare to Live Fully Right Where You Are* (Zondervan, 2011).

Cancer Support:

James R. Kok, *90% Of Helping Is Just Showing Up* (Faith Alive Christian Resources, 1996).

Siddhartha Mukherjee, *The Emperor of All Maladies: A Biography of Cancer* (Scribner, 2010).

Joe E. Pennel, *The Gift of Presence: A Guide to Helping Those Who Suffer* (Abingdon Press, 2009).

Dan Shapiro, *And in Health: A Guide for Couples Facing Cancer Together* (Trumpeter, 2013).

Running:

John L. Parker, *Again to Carthage* (Breakaway Books, 2008).

John L. Parker, *Once a Runner* (Cedarwinds, 1978).

John L. Parker, *Racing the Rain* (Scribner, 2015).

TRAINING, COACHING, CONSULTING, AND SPEAKING SERVICES

For three decades, Mari Martin and PSG have helped organizations optimize the performance of their business, nonprofit, and faith-based teams with versatile training, coaching, and proven expertise in individual development and team dynamics. These services help teams understand how to work together to maximize results, identify the constraints and barriers that get in the way of achieving those results, and minimize stress for everyone when working together.

Our Road Map for Organizational Effectiveness:

1. Discover the Talents to Succeed—develop self-awareness and identify your organization's strengths.
2. Anticipate Conflicts to Contain—recognize work-style differences that create organizational conflict.
3. Pursue Alignment in Assignments—match, hire, and promote team members to the jobs/roles best suited to them.
4. Practice Communication to Connect—adopt common language and principles to work well together and enhance collaboration.
5. Follow the Formula for a High-Performing Team—create healthy, productive, and effective teams that utilize and leverage team members' strengths and work styles.

223

6. Maintain a Commitment to Execute—it's not what you say but what you repeatedly do that counts.

Mari is a Kolbe Certified™ Master Team Consultant and provides the full suite of Kolbe Wisdom™ training, coaching, and consulting services.

To learn more about Mari and PSG Inc., please visit www.psgteam.com, or comehomealivebook.com. If you would like to connect directly with Mari to help you implement any of the concepts in the book or to schedule a speaking engagement, you can call her at PSG (which also stands for People Serving God) 616-219-1356, or email her at mari@psgteam.com.

KOLBE INDEXES

IDENTIFY & LEVERAGE INSTINCTIVE STRENGTHS

Kolbe Corp's proprietary research has shown that our natural creative instincts shape how we accomplish tasks and solve problems in four distinctive behavior patterns, or Action Modes:

- Fact Finder - Ways of gathering and sharing information
- Follow Thru - Ways of organizing
- Quick Start - Ways of dealing with risk and uncertainty
- Implementor - Ways of handling space and tangibles

The first step in the Kolbe System is to determine the instinctive traits within an organization. This is done with the Kolbe A™ Index. The four-number Index result identifies an individual's natural tendencies in each Action Mode and determines his or her modus operandi or MO. The numerical values indicate how a person uses their instincts to prevent problems, respond to opportunities and initiate solutions.

The Kolbe A™ Index
measures and validates a person's natural talents - the instinctive method of operation (MO) that enables you to be your best.

The Kolbe B™ Index
identifies a person's job-related conative self-expectations.

The Kolbe C™ Index
identifies the characteristics a supervisor requires for success in a specific job.

Comparisons: A to A™

How can we work well together?

The Comparisons: A to A™ report provides an analysis of conative Strengths between two individuals with a customized report prepared for each of them.

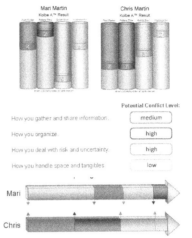

Mari Martin
Kolbe A™ Result

Chris Martin
Kolbe A™ Result

- Ideal for business partners, co-workers or anyone working in tandem on a project
- Analyzes your potential for conative stress
- Identifies what you will do well together and when it's best to work independently
- Conables® tips designed just for you to increase productivity and meaningful communication • Identifies the worst mistake you could make in each of the four Kolbe Action Modes®

Potential Conflict Level:

How you gather and share information.	medium
How you organize.	high
How you deal with risk and uncertainty.	high
How you handle space and tangibles	low

Mari

Chris

Kolbe A™ Index Required.
To learn more about Comparisons: A to A™ or other Kolbe Corp material, visit: ComeHomeAliveBook.com

takes ♈ two

The one thing you need to know to have a better relationship . . .

Let's face it, there isn't "one thing," or a simple "secret" someone can tell you to make your relationships work better. But the good news is that you can learn things about each other that will make it easier to have a stronger, easier, more joyful relationship.

If you're committed to having a great relationship, you need to be committed to extending yourself for the other person.

One indispensable part of that process (and it's a process that continues as long as you're still in that relationship) is understanding each other, and yourselves. That's where Takes Two comes in.

Chris
7 · 7 · 5 · 2

Mari
4 · 2 · 9 · 4

INTRO

First, let's get this straight - we are here to help you figure each other out and give you insight and yes, a little advice about how you can have a better, happier and easier relationship. Yes, you should want your relationship to be 'easier.' That doesn't mean you won't be challenged to grow and evolve, it means not having to struggle to get past what should be small problems. Then you'll have left over energy you can devote to making your relationship even better than you imagined. Maybe you're a workaholic and you just want to have a 'good enough' relationship and put more energy into making your next billion dollars. That's up to you.

So, where were we? . . . Right, insight. And remember, we said some of this is pretty easy. Where do you want to start?

COMMUNICATION

FINANCES

HOUSEHOLD CHORES

VACATIONS

Kolbe A™ Index required.
To learn more about Takes Two® and other Kolbe Corp materials, visit: ComeHomeAliveBook.com

CPSIA information can be obtained
at www.ICGtesting.com
Printed in the USA
LVHW090209190421
684878LV00007B/50